Little Helper

Mummy's
Little Helper

CASEY WATSON

THE HEARTRENDING TRUE STORY OF
A YOUNG GIRL SECRETLY CARING FOR
HER SEVERELY DISABLED MOTHER

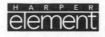

This book is a work of non-fiction based on the author's experiences.
In order to protect privacy, names, identifying characteristics,
dialogue and details have been changed or reconstructed.

HarperElement
An Imprint of HarperCollins*Publishers*
77–85 Fulham Palace Road,
Hammersmith, London W6 8JB

www.harpercollins.co.uk

and *HarperElement* are trademarks of
HarperCollins*Publishers* Ltd

First published by HarperElement 2013

1 3 5 7 9 10 8 6 4 2

A catalogue record of this book is
available from the British Library

ISBN: 978-0-00-747959-7

Printed and bound in Great Britain by
Clays Ltd, St Ives plc

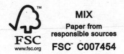

To my wonderful and supportive family

Acknowledgements

I would like to thank all of the team at HarperCollins, the lovely Andrew Lownie, and my friend and mentor, Lynne.

Chapter 1

I love my family. I really do. They're the best in the world in almost every respect. But sometimes they do tend to gang up on me.

'Mum, that's bonkers,' my daughter Riley said, as I brandished the clutch of paint-colour cards I had collected that morning from the local DIY superstore. 'You said it yourself. Trust me, I remember very clearly. You said, "The upstairs is just fine as it is."'

'Perfect,' my husband Mike chipped in pointedly. I glared at him. 'Honest!' he persisted, ignoring it. 'That's what you said, love. That the whole house was perfect. Perfect as it *was*, you said. Remember?'

That was true, certainly. But I chose to pretend I hadn't heard him. Instead I looked at my Kieron, for support. If I could rely on one person at this point, it would be my son. He wouldn't let them browbeat me in this scurrilous fashion, surely? But I was sorely mistaken.

'Come on, you *did*, Mum,' he said, his face a picture of innocence, even as he threw me to the lions. 'And we *did* do the downstairs ...'

'The *whole* of the downstairs,' added Riley. 'And in a *week*. Look. I still have the blisters to prove it!'

I fanned my rainbow of blues and pinks and fixed them all with a steely glare. 'All right then,' I said. 'I'll be the little red hen, then. I shall just have to do it by myself!'

Except I wouldn't. I knew I'd talk them round eventually.

That had been a week back, and true to my prediction I had managed to persuade Mike of the logic of my plan, and with him on board the kids had caved in and helped too. It had been, I'd decided, an inspired idea. With one bedroom for us, and one earmarked for visitors, we had two bedrooms free for our fostering needs. Two bedrooms, to my mind, meant one blue and one pink. That way, I explained to Mike, we'd be always at the ready, whichever gender John Fulshaw sent us next. John Fulshaw was our fostering-agency link worker, and a dear friend. He'd trained us, and had been by our sides ever since.

'Save time and money doing it this way in the long run,' I'd pointed out. And I knew Mike couldn't argue with that. We'd been fostering for four years now and had no thoughts of stopping, so being prepared for anything – and anyone – made sense. Though back at the start, when we'd taken in our first foster child, Justin, I had, I knew, gone slightly overboard. So much so that, when he left us, and our next child was a girl, it was no small task changing our boy's room to a girl's room. I'd gone so mad I'd football themed almost everything in it, right down to the border, the carpet, the clock and the curtains – I'd even painted footballs on the bookcase!

And, as ever, the family rallied round, just as they had this time. It seemed incredible to think we'd been in our new home for barely a month. It was the beginning of February now, and we'd only moved in a couple of days before Christmas. If it hadn't been for everyone pitching in to get the place the way I wanted it – what with the holidays, and having just waved goodbye to our last foster child, Spencer – I felt sure that I wouldn't have felt half as settled as I did.

But, yes, Mike was right, the house *was* perfect. It had been perfect when we'd viewed it, and was even more perfect now. I could barely believe our luck, really. We'd been eighteen years in our last house, and it had been something of a wrench leaving our children's childhood home. There were just so many happy memories wrapped up in it.

And it had been a stressful situation that had prompted it, as well. The move had actually been brought about because of problems with Spencer. He'd been a particularly challenging child to foster, to put it mildly, and his antics (at just eight he'd already been like a one-boy walking crime spree) had caused a lot of upset in the neighbourhood. We weren't exactly forced out, but a great deal of bad feeling had developed, and it had hit home that bringing children such as this into our lives could (and in this case did) have an impact on others, too.

It had certainly forced us to think about the future. And as soon as we'd sat down and considered our options, we realised the timing was right anyway. Not that we'd down-sized. Though our own children had flown the nest (Kieron was settled with his girlfriend Lauren, and Riley and her partner David even had two little ones of their own) we'd moved house with children very much still in mind. Our new place was that little bit further out of town, that bit more open and leafy, that bit more suited to serving our fostering needs.

And now, I thought, as I looked around my two freshly painted bedrooms, the house itself was, as well. Now all I needed was a child to put in one of them.

'So is there anything in the pipeline?' Riley asked me, having admired both the makeovers. It was Tuesday lunch-time, and Levi, my eldest grandson, was back in nursery full time now, so she'd brought baby Jackson over for a sandwich and a natter before going to pick him up. It seemed impossible to me – almost like the blink of an eye – that my first grandson was three now, and that Jackson would be one year old next month.

Impossible but true. Where had all the time gone? I shook my head. 'Not as yet,' I told Riley. 'Though when I spoke to John last week he seemed to think there might be another little boy coming up. With mainstream carers at the moment, but they're apparently struggling to cope with him. Multiple issues,' I went on. 'And some really entrenched disturbing behaviours, by all accounts. John's kind of put us on standby while they decide what to do.'

Riley laughed. 'I bet your ears pricked up straight away,' she commented. 'Multiple issues ... disturbed behaviours ... Sounds right up your street, Mum.'

Which was true; it was exactly why I'd come into fostering. I'd already been thinking about it when I first saw the advertisement for the agency – back when I'd been working as a behaviour manager in a large comprehensive school. An ad seeking people who actively wanted to take on challenging children, the children the system was failing to cope with. 'Fostering the unfosterable' had been the slogan. And it had gripped me straight away. It was what I did at school. It was what I felt I was best at. Oh, yes, I thought, challenging was *right* up my street.

I nodded. 'But that was last week,' I said, as we headed back downstairs. 'I thought I might have heard back by now. I might call him later, as it happens. See what the score is ...'

Riley rolled her eyes. 'You just can't do it, Mum, can you?'

'Do what?' I asked her.

She burst out laughing. 'Do nothing!'

I didn't call John in the end. After all, if he had a child for us he'd have called me about them, wouldn't he? But there was no denying I leapt for my mobile when I heard it buzzing at me the following afternoon. Riley was spot on. I was no good at doing nothing. And since I couldn't take a job

– that was a stipulation for our kind of intense fostering – without a child in, I'd soon be climbing all those freshly painted walls. There was only so much cushion plumping a woman can do and stay sane – even a clean freak like me.

And it wasn't just through lack of an occupation that I was bored. Now we'd moved house, Mike, who was a ware-house manager, had a slightly longer journey to work and back every day, and with us new to the area, filling the day was itself a challenge. I needed to get out and about, make new friends and get to know the neighbours. But all of these things would take time.

It was also still winter, the days short and mostly murky, not really conducive yet to ambling round the neighbour-hood, striking up conversations with strangers. And though our new garden was delighting me almost daily with tanta-lisingly unidentifiable green shoots, I'd never been much of a one for sitting around. I might be a grandma, but I was still only forty-four. A new challenge was exactly what I wanted.

I was in luck. I picked up my mobile to find John's name on the display. 'John,' I said. 'How very nice to hear from you. Are we on?'

'Yes and no,' he said, piquing my interest immediately. 'Though, if you're up for it, it's going to be something of a change of plan.'

'Oh?' I asked, intrigued, pulling out a kitchen chair to sit down. He sounded a little tired and I wondered what he might have been up to. His wasn't an everyday sort of job, for sure.

'Well, if you and Mike are amenable, that is.'

'You already said that,' I said. 'Which sounds ominous in itself.'

'Not at all,' he was quick to correct me. 'Not in the way you probably mean, anyway. I mean as in we're no longer planning on lining you up with that lad we talked about. Got something of an emergency situation on our hands. It's a girl. Nine years old. Rather unusual scenario for us. I've spent most of the day at the General as it happens.'

'The hospital?'

'Yup. Got a call from social services first thing. The mother's quite ill. She has multiple sclerosis –'

'Oh, the poor thing.'

'Yes, the whole situation's pretty grim, frankly. Collapsed this morning, by all accounts, while out trying to buy her daughter a birthday present – she's going to be ten soon. The little girl's called Abigail, by the way – Abby – and she's obviously terribly distraught. Looks like Mum's going to have to be hospitalised for a period. And there is no other family, which means they have no choice but to ...'

'... take her into care?' My heart went out to her. The poor child. Not to mention the poor mother. Having their lives ripped apart so suddenly like this. 'No family at all?' I asked.

'Two second cousins, that's all, both of whom live hundreds of miles away. And they're not remotely close. Never even met the daughter, let alone know her. So it's not workable. The last thing anyone wants is for little Abby to be dragged off somewhere, when Mum's here in hospital, as you can imagine. So she's had a social worker appointed – Bridget Conley. Have you come across her?'

The name was familiar, but I didn't think our paths had yet crossed. But I was more interested in how Mike and I fitted into this. From what John was telling me this was a pretty straightforward scenario. A routine foster placement while a care package was presumably put in place for the mother so that they could both go home. Short term. Crisis management. Not the sort of thing Mike and I were needed for. Our speciality involved long-term placements and a defined behaviour-management programme, and was usually for kids who'd been in the care system a long time already and/or had come from profoundly damaging backgrounds. I said as much to John.

'Ah, well, that's where this isn't quite what you might expect, Casey. The mum's had MS for years. Periods of remission here and there, thankfully, but her condition is quite advanced. The fact that she made it into town at all was something of a miracle, apparently. She's pretty much housebound and quite profoundly disabled ...'

'So how's she been managing to look after her little girl, then? You say there's no family ...'

'Not much of anything or anyone, really, it seems to me. Certainly no care or support in place. She's mentioned a neighbour, but we've already had a clear impression that in terms of who's looked after whom, it's been the other way around. Little Abby's been her carer, pretty much.'

Which was a sobering thought, but still didn't fully answer my question. 'But why us?' I asked again. 'I mean, we're obviously happy to step in, you know that. But if it's only going to be temporary ...'

'It's not going to be *that* temporary,' John corrected me. 'That's what we've been thrashing out today. The medics have given Mum a less than good prognosis, and there's no way in the world they're ever going to discharge a sick patient back to the care of a nine-year-old girl. Bottom line is that even if they manage to get her stable and home, and a package of medical support put in place for her, she's clearly not going to be in a position to care for her daughter, which leaves social services with no choice but to take responsibility for Abby, doesn't it? That's the truth of it. Now the genie's out of the bottle, so to speak ...'

And the cat out of the bag, come to that. John was right, of course. Now they knew about it, they couldn't un-know it. Which left everyone concerned in the worst of all situations. 'God,' I said, as the enormity of it hit home for me. I tried to imagine being told I could no longer look after my own children. Having to watch them being taken away from me, when they needed me. It hardly bore thinking about. 'Poor, poor woman,' I said to John. 'She must be beside herself ...'

'Completely distraught,' John agreed. 'As you can imagine. But not stupid. She knows there's no other choice here.'

'And the poor little girl ... how on earth is she dealing with all this?'

'Badly,' John said. 'Which is where you and Mike come in. Because now we've met her we don't think she's suitable for mainstream care, basically. We've had a long chat with

Mum this afternoon, and she wants what's best for her child, after all.'

'Of course ...'

'And, well, we're all of the opinion that Abby might be, well, how shall I put it? A little idiosyncratic. I must stress that this isn't coming from Mum, before you ask. It's just our assessment, based on what Bridget has seen, and from what we know of how the two of them have been living. I'm obviously not conversant with all the details, but the bottom line would seem to be that this particular nine-year-old is not like any normal nine-year-old. She's been caring for her mum from a very young age, and has basically had no sort of childhood. I know it sounds daft and, yes, we could be over-dramatising this, but our feeling is that being with you and Mike, and doing the programme kind of back to front, if you like, would give her the best chance of getting back on track. You know, getting her used to living as a child again, basically.'

'You've obviously met her,' I said. 'How did she seem to you?'

'Odd, definitely. Twitchy. Has some pronounced – very obvious – tics. I think that's how I'd describe it. Anxious. *Incredibly* anxious. Wound up about as tight as she can be, is my feeling. I mean she's in a state of trauma right now, obviously, but, reading between the lines, there's probably much more besides. So it seemed to us that the best thing would be to take this bull by the horns. Crazy to slot her into a mainstream placement only to have it break down again in a matter of days or weeks.'

'Absolutely,' I agreed, feeling that familiar surge of adrenalin that always accompanied the prospect of a new child. 'Though I hope your faith in us isn't going to be misplaced, John. We're not psychiatrists ...'

'I know. Absolutely. And we'll obviously be reviewing things as a matter of urgency. Counselling's probably a must-do that needs flagging up right away. But I know you two can give her that something extra, in terms of structure, that she probably needs right now.'

'I like to think so. We'll certainly do our best. So. When do you want to schedule a meeting? Just name the day.'

'Ah,' said John. And it was a kind of 'ah' I'd heard from him before. 'That's the thing,' he went on. 'I was wondering if we could skip that part of the process.'

'Ri-ight ...' I said.

'Because I really think we need to bring her now.'

'Ri-ight ...' I said again, waiting for the next part of *this* process. The one where not only did we skip an initial meeting, but also skipped the first 'get to know you a little' visit, which was included to be sure both parties felt happy to proceed. I was fairly confident about this because by now I knew John well.

And he didn't let me down. 'We were kind of hoping you'd agree to take her on right away. If you're amenable, that is ...' he finished apologetically. 'Are you? I know it's a lot to ask.'

I smiled to myself, loving how John always observed all the little protocols, bless him. Because when you thought about it, it wasn't a lot to ask, really, was it? It was the job we did and I couldn't think of a single prior occasion when 'the process', as written in the foster carer's bible, had ever actually happened by the book.

And who cared? Doing things by the book was boring anyway. 'Of course we are,' I reassured him. 'Well, I am, at any rate, and so will Mike be, I'm sure, just as soon as I call and tell him. He'll be glad, to be honest, because it'll give me something else to think about besides all the home improvements he's terrified I'm going to schedule for our already perfect house.'

John laughed. 'So I've actually done him a favour then, have I? Okay, so, let me see … okay if we pitch up in something like an hour and a bit?'

I told him yes, and immediately mentally switched gears. Outside the sun was slinking away from overseeing another grey February day. But suddenly I couldn't care less. I disconnected and immediately reconnected – this time to Mike. I couldn't wait for him to get home. Our New Year had begun.

Chapter 2

Mike was home just in time for us to belt to the local supermarket and stock up with a few supplies before John arrived with our new house guest. On a bit of a New Year health kick, I had little in the way of treats in, and the couple of Christmas biscuits I'd had left in the tin had been hoovered up by Jackson and Riley the day before. It would be a bit of a mad rush, but I was determined to get it done, as I had no idea how things would pan out when Abigail arrived, and wanted to be able to concentrate all my energies on her. On the way I briefed Mike about what I already knew.

'What a dreadful situation,' he said as we parked the car. 'Really makes you count your blessings, doesn't it?' I nodded. 'But, at the same time, it couldn't be better timing for us, could it? Sounds like she's going to be the opposite of Spencer, at least, bless him.'

He was certainly right there. Our last foster child, to use the parlance, had run us ragged. So much so that I think we'd both been holding our breath when we'd been given the all clear two weeks back. Up till then we'd been on standby and unable to take another child, just in case his new situation – back with Mum and Auntie, but not Dad – proved to be unworkable for keeps. He had become so dear to us, and I was looking forward to hearing how he was getting on, but there was no doubt a part of me was warming to the idea of having the novelty (which it would be) of a quiet and well-behaved little girl taking his place. A distressed and anxious one, clearly – and no wonder, given her circumstances – but one with a completely different set of challenges to be overcome.

I grabbed a basket and tried to compile a list in my head of the sort of goodies I thought Abigail might like, getting Mike – six foot three to my own five foot nothing – to reach the items I couldn't. Things didn't normally involve so much guesswork, of course. The usual procedure, as well as those all-important meetings we weren't having, involved the child filling in a short questionnaire we'd devised, in which they could tell us about all their likes and dislikes. It was just one of the ways we could help them feel settled at what was inevitably a stressful and unhappy time in their lives. With everything new and different it could be a comfort for a child to have some constants still in place – be it a favourite snack or special meal, or a much-loved TV programme not missed; such details could make all the difference to a child in distress.

With Abigail, however, we were going in blind, so I just used my judgement to throw in what occurred to me, while

Mike lugged the increasingly heavy basket. 'And at least we have some girl's toys tucked away,' I said, remembering our last little girl, Olivia, who'd come to us from a home of appalling neglect, and owned nothing bar one filthy, balding doll. I'd had something of a field day down at the charity shops for Olivia, and still had a good supply of soft toys and doll's clothes, even if at nine Abigail might be too old for the enormous plastic play kitchen which had been my best-ever find to date.

Mike frowned, though. 'I imagine playing's going to be the last thing on her mind, love,' he pointed out. 'For the moment, at least. Poor kid. She must be reeling.'

He was right, of course. This was a uniquely sad and strange scenario – and for *all* of us. One step at a time. We quickly paid and hurried home.

We'd just finished putting things away and boiling the kettle when John's car pulled up outside. I loved that this new house gave me a window onto the world. My kitchen was at the front of the house this time, and as it was where I spent most of my time it enabled me to indulge in my secret desire to be a 'nosey neighbour'. I also liked the fact that we only had a small front garden. One, better still, that was covered with pebbles, so I wouldn't have to spend much time on maintenance. The other positive was that just across the small road beyond our garden there was a nice grassy area with a children's play section. That was enough to quell any guilt I had about my small but beautifully kept courtyard; that and the fact that we had a rather large back garden that I intended to fill with child-friendly play things for both the grandchildren and the children we'd be fostering.

Abigail looked dwarfed as she walked up the path in between John and her social worker. Still in her green-and-black school uniform, she stole a quick glance at me and Mike as we opened the front door. She was a pretty little girl, slim and petite, with her long fair hair held in two bunches which were neatly tied with matching green ribbon.

She also looked terrified. I was used to greeting children in distress, of course. There can be few things more bewildering and disorientating for a child than being made to go and live with complete strangers. But most children who came into foster care did so in carefully managed stages, so that even if the process was, by its nature, a relatively quick one, by the time it came to actually being deposited with their temporary family, the child had at least been there for a visit.

Poor Abby had had no such preparation. In less than a day her whole life had imploded. She'd gone to school this morning fully expecting to go home again and instead, she'd been picked up and told her mother was ill in hospital and that tonight she would have to sleep somewhere else. I was used to dealing with kids from bad family situations, but it still seemed inexplicable to me that this sweet little girl didn't have a single other place she could go to. When my own two were her age it would have been unthinkable. Riley had her little gang of sleepover mates, most of whose mums were friends of mine too. All would have stepped in during a crisis like this one, just as I'd have stepped in had it been them.

My thoughts also naturally went to my Kieron, and how he would have fared in such a crisis. He was all grown up now – twenty-two – but he had Asperger's Syndrome, a mild type of autism. He functioned well, had been to college and was doing well in life, but a change – any change – to his routine really stressed him. For someone like him, such a thing would be a major trauma. I'd thanked God many times for my network of friends and family, who knew his needs and idiosyncrasies and so could always help de-stress him. How would I have ever coped without them over the years?

Yet for this poor little girl there was no one. The social worker had already questioned both Abby and her mum about this, thinking, quite rightly, that if no family could be found at short notice, then a sleepover with a close pal would be the very next best thing. But no, it seemed the child didn't have anywhere else to go. Unbelievable. And what on earth must have been going through her mind, knowing not only that complete strangers were rearranging her whole future, but that she had to go and live with some, too? I could only hope that the enormity of what might happen long term hadn't yet impinged on her consciousness. As far as I was concerned, the best way to manage her in the short term would be to focus very much on the here and now.

I smiled my broadest smile as she hesitantly stepped into the hallway. Both her hands gripped the straps of the backpack she was carrying, and so tightly that the knuckles were white. I smiled as I recognised the logo on the backpack: 'Glee', accompanied by the all-singing, all-dancing cast publicity photo. Straight away I was thinking that if Abby liked all the latest stage-school TV programmes and paraphernalia, she would get along famously with Lauren. Lauren was Kieron's girlfriend and was at performing arts college, and was used to me roping her in to help out with similarly minded foster children.

I also recognised the primary-school logo on Abby's sweatshirt. Stanholme Primary, although the furthest away, was one of the better schools in the area, and also a feeder school for the big comprehensive I used to work at, and I'd known a couple of the teachers there. It was good to have a pre-existing connection with the place. It gave me a head start in that direction, at least.

'Here she is. Here's Abigail!' John said, with a slightly forced brightness – he looked as worn out as he'd sounded on the phone. I ushered the trio into the dining room and Mike took their orders for hot drinks. Not that he had to go far to make them; like our last house, this too had an open-plan kitchen/dining set-up, the only difference being that the two were separated by a huge arch. Perfect, once again, for keeping an eye on kids.

Right now, of course, I had my eyes on Abigail. She'd hardly spoken – only mumbled an affirmative to a hot chocolate – and looked completely at sea, as if she might burst into tears or make a run for it at any moment. Again, this felt so different from what we'd seen before. We might be strangers – as might be John – but all our previous children had come to us with at least some sort of relationship, however slight, with the social worker assigned to them. As a result they usually clung to them, both physically and emotionally. But that was definitely not the case here.

Bridget Conley, a tall woman in her early forties, I guessed, filed in behind John. She looked nice enough, if a little detached, but it was so immediately obvious she and Abigail had barely met. It would have been so even if I hadn't already known that. No one's fault – all this had happened in less than a day, after all – though I couldn't help feeling it a pity that they hadn't managed to make some sort of connection. Bridget (whose face was vaguely familiar to me, nothing more) looked friendly and personable, but also as if she'd come from the sort of high-level meeting that she'd felt the need to power-dress for that morning. Where social workers normally dressed to suit the work they did – in comfortable, non-threatening, relaxed clothes, in my experience – Bridget looked more like a head teacher or a politician: all sharp angles, crisp creases and clacky shoes.

And I'd been right. 'Apologies,' she began as she started fishing in a laptop bag. 'I'm not at all up on the paperwork, I'm afraid.' She grimaced. 'Been attending a case conference with my manager and her boss. Hence the suit and heels, I'm afraid.' She grinned, somewhat sheepishly. 'Why on earth do these things always get me so flustered? You'd think with twenty years in the job I'd be a little less bothered about dressing up for the upper echelons, wouldn't you?' She laughed then, and I found myself warming to her. A woman very much like myself, I thought.

John, too, was pulling the inevitable manila file from his briefcase, with such scant notes as he'd presumably been so far able to make. And looking at the tableau of officialdom in front of me made me have something of a 'eureka!' moment. While Mike clattered with cups and teaspoons, I looked straight at John. 'I tell you what,' I said to him. 'How about you all take a breather for a moment and enjoy a cup of tea. Been quite a long and stressful day, eh?' I said, turning my gaze now to Abigail. 'And why don't you and I take a look round my beautiful new garden? We've only just moved in here, and I'm so excited about it. And it'll be dark soon ...' I held out my hand.

My hunch had been right. No sooner had Abigail seen it than she'd grabbed hold of it gratefully and, finally being persuaded to take off the backpack, she let me lead her from the room. It was if she'd been drowning and was desperate for a life-belt to cling on to; an escape from the turbulent waters of this surreal situation that she had suddenly, inexplicably found herself in.

I led her through the living room and pulled open the French doors that looked out onto the garden. 'How about that, then?' I asked her.

I watched her gaze go exactly where I'd imagined it would – to the enormous trampoline in the far corner. It had been something we'd inherited – literally – as we'd been told the previous tenants, who'd gone abroad, had had no time to dismantle it and sell it. So they'd simply left it for whoever moved into the house next, much to Levi and Jackson's delight. 'It's a big one, isn't it?' I added, smiling down at Abby now.

She dutifully smiled back and stepped outside with me into the garden. 'You know, I have two little grandsons, Abigail. There's Levi, who's three, and baby Jackson, who's nearly one. If you like, when they come to play you could show them how to bounce on it.'

Abigail, who was still clutching my hand, looked thoughtful. 'Yes, I'd like that,' she said, sounding almost painfully solemn. 'But Mrs Watson? I think you need to put a net around it first. I've seen them on TV and you need those for very little people.'

Bless her, I thought, touched by her serious tone. 'You know what?' I said. 'You're right. And I never thought about that, love. I'll have to mention it to Mike, won't I? Good point. By the way, do you prefer to be called Abigail or Abby?'

Again, she seemed to need to think carefully before answering. 'Well, my mummy calls me Abby, so I think I'd prefer that. Though my teachers call me Abigail, so I don't suppose it matters. Whichever you want, really.'

She looked up at me, managed to find another half-smile from somewhere. 'No contest, then,' I said. 'Abby it is.'

She didn't seem to know what to do or say then, and seemed content to let me lead her on a short tour of the garden, while I did the bulk of the talking. Now clearly wasn't the time to expect her to open up to me. She'd probably been bombarded with questions from the minute she'd been fetched from school and taken to the hospital. And I didn't doubt her mind was very much still back there, with her poor mum. My heart went out to her. She must have felt as if she'd been abducted by aliens, which, in a practical sense, she sort of had. What I imagined she most needed was a distraction from the clamour of her fearful thoughts. 'So,' I told her, 'I'm called Casey, okay? No "Mrs Watson". And Mike, that great big man you just met in there? Well, he's my husband. And what we do is look after children who, for whatever reason, can't stay in their own homes for a bit. Did John explain all that to you? Why you're here?'

Abigail nodded. It was growing dark now and I led us across to the bench seat on the patio. It was cold, but not wet, as it was partly sheltered by a fibre-glass lean-to. It was the only disappointment; a poor second to the wonderful conservatory we'd had in the last house. But it was functional, at least. And also temporary. Mike didn't know it, but I fully intended to wait a few months, and then badger him mercilessly about getting us a new one. I patted the space beside me on the bench, and she obediently sat down, finally letting go of my hand.

'So that's what we're going to do,' I went on. 'Take care of you. So you mustn't worry about anything, okay? And the first thing we're going to do is get things sorted so we can get you back to visit your mum as soon as possible –'

'Tonight?' she asked timidly. 'I really need to make sure she's okay.'

I shook my head. 'Not tonight, I don't think,' I said gently. 'But definitely this week. If not tomorrow, the next day. After school. We'll make sure of that, don't worry.

We'll fix it up with John and Bridget, before they go. And Mummy'll be fine, you know. She's in a safe place, and they'll take really good care of her, just like we're going to take really good care of you. Now then, how about that hot chocolate and a biscuit? They'll be wondering where we've got to out here, won't they? Hmm?'

I turned now, to look at her properly. The outside light had already picked out a shiny trail on her face, which marked where tears were slipping silently down her cheeks. The instinctive thing to do, as had been the case with holding out a hand to her, was to pull her towards me and hug her. It was as natural to me as breathing, as it would be to anyone. But with kids in care – particularly the long-term emotionally damaged kids we mostly dealt with – often that's the last thing they need or want. Starved of normal human relationships, or, sometimes, all too familiar with dangerously inappropriate ones, they can find it almost impossible to empathise or be physical with the very people who most want to help them. But this was not that; this was a normal and clearly much-cherished little girl, who wanted nothing more keenly to be back with the mum who loved her. I scooped her into my arms and she sobbed hard against my chest, and as she did so I reflected that some good might come of this. Fingers crossed, they would soon sort out something workable for her mum's care and, that done, she'd be able to enjoy at least some semblance of normality for what still remained of her childhood.

I had no reason to expect things to be otherwise at that point. Silly me. Is life ever that simple?

Chapter 3

Abby seemed much better for a cry and a cuddle, and when we returned to the dining room she had got herself composed again, and settled down to a biscuit and her by now lukewarm hot chocolate, which she wouldn't let Mike pop into the microwave for her. 'It's safer to drink it like this, anyway,' she said quietly, before wrapping both her hands around the mug.

'So,' said John, once he'd confirmed details of the hospital visit and reassured Abby that she'd soon be able to see her mum again. 'I think we're about done here. And I expect this little lady needs to get to bed, eh?' He looked at Abby, who was staring into her now empty mug as if it might hold the answer to how she had come to be here. She looked up at him, as if the word 'bed' was physically painful. All she wanted, I felt sure, was her *own* bed.

Mike and I exchanged glances while Bridget said her goodbyes. The mood was sombre now, Bridget having outlined, albeit in the gentlest of tones, that for the moment, at least, Abby would only be able to visit her mum a couple of times a week. Though I understood why – daily visits would be both impractical (the hospital was some distance away) and could potentially slow down the process of adjustment – I really felt for her. This was the mum she had seen every single day for her entire life. No wonder she looked so distraught.

And to really hammer home the drastic and abrupt nature of this disaster, here she was, being deposited with us – a pair of strangers. We were used to this, of course – this business of children who hardly knew us being delivered to our doorstep – but we really *were* strangers to Abby. No preliminary visits, no chance to get used to the idea; I kept reminding myself that she'd first clapped eyes on us less than an hour ago. I also tried to keep in mind that in the Second World War this was something that hundreds of thousands of kids had gone through, my own and Mike's parents included. But that was a lifetime away, and knowing it would be of absolutely no comfort to this traumatised child. I stood up again and went round to her side of the table. 'I thought we might have a little sit-down together before bed,' I said, placing my hands on her shoulders and dipping my head close to hers. 'Once we've shown you your bedroom and you've unpacked and we've had our tea, of course. And a rummage through my special bits and bobs box, as well. I had this idea. I thought it might be an idea to get a bit of a diary started. Even a scrapbook, perhaps, that we can stick pictures and special things into.

So you can keep mummy up to date with what you get up to while you're here. Would that be an idea? I bet she'd like that, don't you?'

I could once more see the white of Abby's knuckles as she held on to the mug. She was close to tears again, I noticed, now John and Bridget were leaving. For all that there hadn't been time for them to forge a bond yet, Bridget's was obviously still the most familiar face in the room.

And Bridget could clearly see that herself. She wasn't stupid; she knew that to gush at Abby now would create a chink in her fragile composure. Like every social worker, I imagined she'd had her fair share of situations where a desperate child had clung on to her for grim death. 'Splendid!' she declared briskly, as she shrugged on her jacket and slid her slim sheaf of papers back into their slipcase. 'And when I'm back –' She glanced at me now. 'Which will be in – let me see now … two weeks – you can show me all the things you've been up to with Mike and Casey, hmm? All the adventures you've been having with them. Yes?'

Poor Bridget. Abby looked positively mortified by this. As well she might have. She'd already had so much 'adventure' in this one day that I felt sure the principal thought going through her mind right then was that even one more adventure would be one too many.

* * *

Abby had come to us with a small, carefully packed suitcase, which would have been collected from home after she'd been picked up from school by the on-duty social worker. By this time they would already have put the wheels in motion, so that John could sort an emergency placement, i.e. us. It was a well-oiled machine, social services, in this regard, but for Abby it must have been terrifying.

I sat on the bed and watched as she carefully began taking out the contents, having opened the dresser drawers ready. The case was full. It contained another set of school uniform, a small pile of neatly folded clothes, plus pyjamas, socks and pants, a pink toothbrush and a doll. As she went methodically through the contents, I wondered who'd packed it, then rolled my eyes at my own stupidity. *She* would have done it; who else? She was used to doing everything for herself, wasn't she? I made a point of not fussing too much about helping her put things away; she seemed to have a very set way of doing everything, and I could see she was also double checking everything as she did it: she put socks in a drawer, closed it, then opened it again to check, and only then moved on to the next task, which she'd do similarly. It was odd, but I decided to let her get on with it; interfering would probably only make her more anxious than she already was.

'That's a pretty doll,' I said instead, as she took out the last couple of items, which were an equally carefully packed set of doll's clothes. The doll herself – which was a large one, with long blonde wavy hair, much like her own – was currently dressed as a mermaid. The other outfits, I could see, were also mermaid ones, and quite elaborate; one was decorated with tiny pink feathers, and the other, blue sequins. The doll was clearly much loved, and taken very good care of – a world away from the scant possessions most of our foster kids arrived with. Abby propped her against the pillows and smoothed her hair.

'She's called Ariel,' she told me. 'Aren't you, Ariel?'

'Well, hello, Ariel,' I said. 'Very pleased to meet you. But, gosh, look at the time. It's getting late, isn't it?' I stood up to draw the pink-and-purple butterfly-print curtains and flick the switch on the matching bedside lamp. They'd been a real find on eBay – my latest stuff-procurement hobby – and a great asset to my foster-bedroom decorating plans. The room looked cosy and welcoming, at least. 'Way past teatime, in fact,' I added. 'Mike'll be starving. Are you hungry?'

Poor Mike would, too, I thought, wondering if he was rummaging in the kitchen cupboards as I spoke. I'd left him downstairs washing up the cups and saucers. But Abby shook her head. 'Not even a little,' she said. 'We had some food at the hospital. I don't really feel like eating anything else, if that's okay.'

'Of course,' I reassured her, remembering the hot chocolate. She'd left the biscuit, but a mug of milky chocolate was pretty filling in itself. And it was gone seven now. I could always make her a sandwich later, if she wanted one. I said so. 'Here, let's have that,' I added, gesturing to the now empty suitcase. 'I'll pop it on the top of the wardrobe for you.'

'But will they make tea for Mummy?' she wanted to know, as she placed her pyjamas on the pillow beside the doll and carefully smoothed the duvet cover where the case had rucked it up.

'What, the hospital? Of *course* they will.'

'They won't forget about her, will they?'

I shook my head. 'Why would they forget about her?'

Abby didn't look convinced. 'If she's sleeping, they might. She needs her sleep. And if she's asleep they might forget her, mightn't they?' She was nibbling the skin around her fingers and talking through them, and I had to stop myself from automatically reaching across and gently pulling her hands from her mouth. Instead, I filed it away for a conversation to have another day. As a child Kieron had always been a great one for nibbling his fingers, and occasionally still did it even now. And with his Asperger's, it was also one of the signs we would look out for. An intense bout of whittling his fingernails to the quick was a sure sign that, even if outwardly he seemed to be coping, inside he most definitely was not.

'Sweetheart,' I told Abby, 'you absolutely mustn't worry. They have a system in hospitals, about food and when they bring it, and if a patient is sleeping they *always* make a note to come back and offer them something later on.'

'But what if they don't? I mean, they might not. They might forget. They have so many patients to look after.'

'They won't forget,' I said. 'Promise. They check every patient regularly. There will be a nurse nearby every single hour of every day.' I pulled the bedroom door open wider.

'Now, then, how about we go down and get that box out, and see what we've got? I was thinking that perhaps we could go on the internet and find some pictures to print out. You could have the cast of *Glee* on the cover of it, perhaps. Something like that.'

Abby nodded, seemingly mollified, and produced a small smile which I hope betrayed at least a spark of enthusiasm. 'Okay,' she said, as I turned to lead the way back downstairs.

Before following me, however, she crossed the bedroom and carefully turned off the bedside lamp, then reached up and flipped the switch for the main light, as well. And then, as we crossed it, she turned off the landing light too. Then on again, as if undecided, and then off again. 'Oh, don't worry,' I began as we were plunged back into near blackness. 'We usually leave that one till we've gone up to bed.'

She turned to face me, her expression one of complete consternation.

'But what about the bills?' she asked incredulously.

It seemed that bills, and the worry of them, not to mention that of timetables for everything from laundry to medication, were what took up most of this small girl's time. After we'd spent a focused half-hour gathering the raw materials for her new scrapbook, I suggested she go up and change into her pyjamas and that we could then watch some TV before she went to bed. We'd abandoned hope of having our usual meal and Mike contented himself with a couple of extra biscuits, the plan being, since Abby still had no interest in dinner, that we'd order in a take-away to eat once she'd gone to bed. It wasn't the usual thing we'd do on a random Tuesday evening, but this, of course, wasn't a usual sort of day.

She'd come back down now and we'd tried to find out a little more about her. There was no point in setting up a tailored behaviour modification programme till we had more idea both about the small person for whom we'd tailor it and the behaviours which most needed modifying.

And it soon became clear – just as John had warned us – that whatever behaviours were worrying social services, they were the result of a life dominated by caring for her mother.

'So what sort of things do you and your friends like doing?' Mike asked her, as we settled in the living room. Abby had gone straight to the big new recliner armchair by the fireplace. It had been a moving-in extravagance, and was already Mike's favourite – but tonight he'd had to come and join me on the sofa. Not that he didn't often, but I smiled even so. After a long day at the warehouse he liked nothing better than to press the button that made the foot-rest pop out, and more often than not declare, 'Fit for a king, this!'

But I knew he didn't mind, bless him. There was a David Attenborough wildlife programme coming on shortly, which we'd both been keen to see, and which Abby had expressed interest in watching too. Her mum, she explained, had really liked the series about the sea – when 'she could still actually see the telly,' she'd added sadly.

She turned to Mike now. 'I don't really have many friends,' she told him, one hand twiddling a few strands of her hair round and round. 'I don't have much time for things like that.'

Mike raised his eyebrows. 'What, none?' he asked, mock-incredulously. 'Not even one special best friend for ever? A BFF – isn't that what they call them these days?'

Abby shook her head. 'Not really,' she repeated, with a shrug. I watched her carefully, but she didn't seem to be distressed making this admission – simply stating a fact. 'I don't need friends anyway,' she added quietly. 'I have Mummy.'

'And a very busy life, by the sound of it,' I said quickly, anxious that she didn't get upset again. Which she clearly was. She was twiddling her hair even faster, though she didn't seem conscious of the fact. 'Oh, and look, the programme's starting,' I said, glad of a distraction for the poor child. 'We've been looking forward to seeing this all week.'

And it was good, too, except I kept getting distracted by Abby who, though her eyes were on the television, seemed in some sort of trance, and continued to play constantly with her hair. As I kept glancing at her, I realised she was no longer playing with a lock of hair, but with single strands, which she'd carefully separate out, using both hands, then wind around her index finger, as you might roll cotton around a pencil, then, with a tiny jerk, pull from her head.

Again and again this would happen – it was almost cease-less. She'd get hold of a strand of hair, spool it slowly up, then – tug – she'd have freed it, whereupon she'd uncoil it and then let it spring free from her finger. Even at a distance of several feet across the room, I could see a tiny nest of hairs growing on the chair arm. And even with the experience of many deeply distressed children, I could see I was dealing with something different here. John had alluded to 'behaviours', but this was new territory. I would definitely have to read up on what we might potentially be dealing with. And definitely not forget about that sandwich.

Chapter 4

John called at nine, as he'd promised he would the night before, for an update on how things had gone. But it was John, not me, who had the most to say in terms of updating, having just returned to his office from a further trip to Abby's home.

In the next few days, assuming Abby's mum remained in hospital, she'd be allocated to a health-care team, who'd take charge of things at home for her, but as a stop-gap it had fallen to Bridget. So John had gone and met her there first thing. Abby's mum, who was apparently called Sarah, had been anxious about the place being empty, and had requested that she go back to check things, make sure the heating had been set to low, and that the windows were all locked, as well as to collect a list of further items for Abby – school books and footwear and her winter coat and so on – none of which, in the rush, she'd had time to take with her, and about which both mother and daughter had been fretting.

'So it made sense for me to take them,' John explained. 'Since I'd be the next one stopping by at yours. So I'll bring them up when I come to you next week. And I am so glad I did go, I can tell you, because it's given me a really useful insight. Just incredible. You'd have to see it to believe it, trust me. It's told us volumes in terms of how these two have been living. It's no wonder they were under the radar. Honestly, Casey, if an alien came to earth on a reconnaissance mission, they'd have everything they needed in that one house alone. There is an instruction for absolutely *everything*. Anyway, first up, how has Abby been overnight? Okay?'

I told him about the hair pulling, and that it was something I'd keep an eye on, but reassured him that, all things considered, she'd been fine. She'd been fast asleep the couple of times I'd gone in and checked on her, and had woken looking marginally less traumatised at least. Though not for long – not once she'd remembered about school.

A taxi had been organised the day before, to take her, and had arrived promptly at eight, its exhaust billowing white in the cold air. It had struck me as a little odd that she'd be going to school at all, but, as Bridget had pointed out, it was important that Abby had at least some normality to cling on to. Besides, it was a special day – it was Abby's class assembly, which was as good a reason as any not to miss it.

But, despite apparently accepting this at the hospital the day before, she'd been upset by its arrival, when the reality of actually going to school sunk in. Not because she was anxious about being there, particularly, but because she was so anxious about her mother's welfare. 'But what about Mummy's breakfast?' she'd asked me, her chin wobbling, as I'd tried to coax her into eating some of her own. I'd gently reminded her that the nurses would have seen to it she had breakfast. 'But what if they don't?' she persisted. 'Or what if they don't know what she likes?'

I'd sat down and explained about the little menu cards for meals they had in hospitals and how patients could tick boxes to say what they wanted, be it porridge, Weetabix or toast and marmalade and so on. But this just threw up another whole set of problems. 'But she won't be able to read it. Will they realise that?' she asked plaintively. 'Will they just think she can and then get cross when she hasn't ticked things?'

I told her no, they certainly wouldn't get cross about *anything*. And that they knew about her mum's MS and how reading was a bit difficult, and reassured her that someone would go through the list *with* her. Which, along with my promise to ring the hospital while she was at school, seemed to settle her enough for her to sit at the kitchen table, at least.

'But then there were the bins,' I explained to John now.

'The bins?' he asked. 'What bins?'

'The bins at her house. Wednesday is dustbin day where they live, apparently. And she was really worried about who would take the bins out for them.'

'Ah,' John said. 'Well, you can certainly reassure her on that point. We've seen the next-door neighbours – the ones on the right, anyway. The house the other side is currently empty – and they've given us a number, in case we need to get in touch with them. I'm hoping that when we next have contact with Sarah we'll be able to persuade her to give them a key as well. I'll ring them if you like; ask them to deal with the bins. That way you can at least put the poor girl's mind at rest.'

'That would be good, John. Because you know what she did, before she left for school?'

'Tell me.'

'She was just about to get into the taxi when she turned around and ran back – I actually thought she'd decided she wasn't going at this point, of course – but, no. She grabbed our wheelie bin and dragged it to the pavement.'

'*Your* wheelie bin? Why would she put out *your* wheelie bin?'

'I know. And I'd already told her it wasn't our bin day. But then I realised she probably just *had* to do it, didn't she? She just couldn't bear to get in that taxi *without* doing it. Would probably have fretted about it all day.'

'Bless her,' said John. 'That's exactly the kind of thing we thought might be a problem. And it's no surprise, frankly, given what Bridget and I have seen this morning. Really brings it home to you how things have been for the poor girl.'

John went on to describe what he'd found at the family home, which was as much of an eye-opener as he'd promised. The whole house, he explained, had been totally modified for a young child to do absolutely everything.

There were sticky notes everywhere – some recent, some old and yellowing – on which were hand-written instructions for doing just about everything you could think of. How to operate the washing machine, how to set the timer and the thermostats for the heating and hot water, how to operate the cooker, the microwave and the grill. There were notes on what temperature setting to use for the fridge – summer and winter – and an inventory of the contents of all the drawers and the cupboards, including crockery and cutlery, pots, pans and bakeware, glasses and mugs, housewares and food. The kitchen also contained evidence of just how much routine there was here. There was a big wall chart, detailing what meals would be eaten and when, and a ring binder, chock full of simple recipes, many of which had been painstakingly written out in a child's handwriting, while others had been torn from magazines.

Abigail also had her own little dedicated cleaning cupboard, where on the inside of the door was written a long list of chores and when to do them: polish wooden furniture and banisters Mondays, bleach in toilet daily, white wash on Thursday, and so on. The house was also liberally strewn with small coloured plastic steps, some of the type you'd use when toilet training a toddler, others larger – including one four-foot stepladder, even – to provide access to high-mounted cupboards.

'Everything you could think of,' John finished. 'Simply everything. Right down to a light-bulb inventory and book of money-off coupons – all in sections – one for each supermarket nearby. If it needs organising, basically, it's been organised into the ground. Never seen anything quite like it in my life. I suspect there's not been a minute of a single day that doesn't – well, *didn't* – come with its own list of jobs. Boot camp. That's the word. It's just like boot camp. Quite remarkable.'

'What was the mother thinking?' I wondered, trying to put myself in her shoes. 'Why on earth didn't she get them some help?'

'Exactly,' John said. 'That's what Bridget and I were both stumped by. I mean, it's hardly as if help for these sorts of things isn't publicised, is it? Couple of clicks of a mouse would have her straight to the MS website, wouldn't it?'

'So did Bridget talk to her about that?'

'A little, she says, though none of it was particularly enlightening. She just said they always managed by themselves, pretty much. Which I can *sort* of see, I suppose. If you're fairly isolated, anyway. Because it's obviously happened gradually – as has the progression of the disease, of course. So I suppose I can see how it's just become their version of "normal". And Abby will never have known any different, will she? Though, that said, she must surely have seen the way other families work, mustn't she? When she's gone to friends' houses for tea and so on – *something* must have clicked.'

'I'm not sure she's done a great deal of that sort of thing,' I told him. 'According to her, she has no friends. Hasn't got the time for them.'

'Well, that *does* ring true,' he said, 'given what we've seen this morning. Anyway, we might find out a little more about all that later on today. Bridget wasn't first on the scene, of course – it was the on-duty social worker … So she's going to chase that up when whoever it was is back in the office later. See if she can find out any more about what's been discussed. But it's certainly odd, isn't it? To cut yourself off from help in that way. Though right now the most pressing thing is to try to find some family. It seems incredible that there's absolutely *no one* who could help.'

'I'll obviously see what I can find out from Abby, too,' I said. 'Maybe she can throw a bit more light on things.'

'That would be helpful. Anyway, the main thing right now is for you to make sure she's okay. From what I've seen this morning, it's no wonder she has anxiety-related issues. Her whole life seems to have been one long to-do list, so some emotional fall-out's going to be expected, isn't it? She's going to find the loss of control hard to adjust to, I'm sure.'

John was right, of course. Abby was dropped home from school and the very first thing she did when I opened the front door to her was to go 'brrr', and ask me where the central heating controls were. Mindful of my discussion with John earlier I simply took her upstairs and showed her, as she had such a pinched, anxious look on her face, that it was clear this was something that had been on her mind for a while.

'Can I have a look?' she asked me, once we were upstairs and peering into the airing cupboard. The controls were set high on the wall, and it was difficult for her to see them.

She was a tiny little thing for her age – a good six inches shorter than Spencer, who'd just left us, even though she was a good year older than him.

'Of course,' I said, spreading my arms. 'Shall I pick you up so you can see?'

She seemed to consider for a moment. As I'm sure I would have done, in her shoes. But her need to know soon seemed to triumph over her shyness. She raised her own arms so I could get my hands under her armpits and lift her up.

As soon as the control panel was at eye level I heard – and felt – her sigh. 'You've got this set too late,' she said, tapping the panel with a finger.

'Have I?' I asked her, as I let her back down to the floor. Despite the gravity of the situation, this was such a surreal moment that I struggled to keep the smile off my face.

Her own expression was deadly serious. 'It's winter,' she pointed out. 'So what I expect you've probably done is forget about the clocks having gone back, when you moved in. Did you check it? Because I think it's set to come on an hour too late.'

I couldn't help but be impressed by her logic. That and the fact that she'd remembered that we'd not long moved in. 'Are you cold?' I asked her, because despite that I wasn't really sure why it was bothering her anyway. I certainly wasn't cold. I rarely was. I went at my domestic chores with far too much energy to feel chilly.

Abby shook her head. 'No, no, not me,' she explained. 'I'm at school all day, aren't I? It's *you*. This really needs to come on at around three o'clock.'

There wasn't much to say to that really, other than that I wasn't cold, and only tended to put the heating on before teatime if I had my little grandsons round and it was a particularly cold day. Which I did, but as soon as I'd done so, and explained that it was obviously different for her mum – she would feel the cold, of course – she seemed even more agitated than she'd been in the first place.

So when we came back downstairs – after she'd changed out of her uniform, and also changed her dolly – I decided I would just go with the flow. Which I'd clearly need to. As soon as I wondered out loud what we could have for tea, she was once again looking stressed and asking questions.

'Don't you know what you're cooking tonight?' she asked me. 'Don't you have a chart?'

'No, sweetheart,' I explained, remembering what John had told me earlier. 'Not really. I mean, I do have a rough plan – some things to choose from. But I generally see what I've got in the fridge and cupboards, then just cook what we most fancy having.'

I was reminded then of Justin, our first foster child. Compared to Abby, his background couldn't have been more different. A veteran – aged only eleven – of twenty failed placements (foster homes and children's homes), he'd come to us in such a state of emotional distress and anger that there had been times when Mike and I had despaired of ever being able to even reach him, let alone do anything to help him.

Abby was so different, on so many levels, yet it seemed we had exactly the same issue in the kitchen; that, like Justin, she needed a very clear set of rules – to know, as he had, exactly what we were eating on which day, and when. So, in terms of strategy, perhaps they weren't going to be so different after all. At least, not in this respect. I smiled at her.

'But now you're here,' I said to her, 'I'm happy to do things your way – it will be such a treat not to have to think what to cook, I can tell you. So. What would *you* like for tea?'

This seemed to be exactly the right thing to say because she immediately looked happier, putting a finger to her lips, and tapping them as she consulted the chart she obviously had in her head.

'Well,' she said, 'it's Wednesday, which is normally scrambled eggs and beans on toast day. If … um … that's all right with you,' she added politely.

'Of course it is,' I told her. 'I've got plenty of both.' I was just about to add that she could help me make it if she liked when she rolled up the sleeves of the hoodie she'd changed into. 'Right,' she said brightly. 'I'll get started, then.'

Of course, one of the things I was aware was in our brief was to gently re-train her to accept that she was a child and, as such, needed to reclaim a childhood. Which obviously meant accepting the normal child–adult roles, which, on the evidence of her first twenty-four hours in our company, was going to be something of a challenge.

But it was early days, so I decided I would let her have a degree of autonomy. For today at least. I told her we would prepare everything and cook it together, ready for when Mike got home from work.

'And you should have seen her,' I told Mike, after we'd finished our tea and I had the chance of a quiet few minutes upstairs with him, while Abby sat and wrote in her new scrapbook. 'There was nothing she couldn't do. She knew how to crack the eggs, whisk them, open the bean tins, and use the correct bowl for them, work out the microwave – absolutely everything.'

Mike grinned. 'And it tasted good too! Sounds like we've lucked out with this one,' he joked. 'A dream, by the sounds of it, certainly compared with young Spencer! More like a housekeeper than a foster child, given half a chance!'

It obviously *was* a joke, and she certainly wouldn't be *given* that half a chance, but even so, I was struggling to see where the challenge in this challenging child lay. Yes, she would have all sorts to deal with in the coming weeks, but compared with the sort of kids we usually looked after, this just didn't seem to be even on the same scale.

But as later that evening we sat and watched her pulling strands of hair out again, a part of me – the rational part – knew better. She was also, we noticed, clock watching – or watch-watching, more accurately. Checking the little pink watch on her wrist again and again and again; looking at it, tapping the face, then pulling her sleeve back over it, then looking and tapping and covering it again. What she was watching for, what precise timing was being monitored, we didn't know: when I asked why – if there was something she needed to remember to do – she coloured. Yet she continued to do it, right until the time she went to bed.

No. I knew better. However benign, compared with other kids', her problems seemed to me, she was with us for a reason, as John had pointed out.

And we'd find out the extent of it soon enough.

Chapter 5

The visit to see Sarah, Abby's mother, had been arranged for around four the following afternoon and, having seen Abby off to school, I spent much of the day wondering what I was going to find when I met her.

Meeting family members in my role as a foster carer was something I'd learned I could never second-guess. It was such a singular and unnatural situation. In some circumstances, of course, you never got to meet the birth parents of a child you cared for, because all contact had been stopped by social services. Other times the relationship was civil, even if tense. Sometimes a parent was angry and downright hostile – we'd had a baptism of fire in that regard, for sure.

You never knew what to expect. Each situation was different. I'd been sworn at, I'd been threatened, I'd been genuinely scared, often, but the experience that had left the most lasting impression had been a couple of years back, with our second foster-child, Sophia, who had come to us after her mother had fallen down the stairs, and ended up in hospital, in a coma.

Like Sarah, Sophia's mother had been on her own, with very little in the way of family, which was why Sophia, after a period of being looked after by an uncle, had finally had to come into care. Visits to Sophia's mother, by the time she had come to live with us, meant visits to a room in a hospice. She was on a life-support system, in a persistent vegetative state, and seeing her for the first time was profoundly shocking. She was so beautiful, and so young, like a sleeping Disney princess. It was an experience I would never forget.

I wasn't expecting anything quite so dramatic – or, indeed, distressing – today. In fact I was looking forward to meeting Sarah. Most kids are in care because they can't be left with their families, more often than not because the families in question were unfit, for whatever reason, to care for them.

This was different. Sarah clearly loved her daughter. It was just cruel fate that had conspired against the pair of them. It was frustrating, certainly, that she'd felt unable to ask for help up to now – and the results of her over-reliance on her little girl were obviously a problem – but who was I to say I wouldn't have done the same in her situation?

And perhaps the illness had crept up on her – multiple sclerosis was like that, wasn't it? And the situation at home – the way everything had been arranged for Abby to do everything – had obviously grown up over a number of years. And if I knew anything about anything it was that if a situation developed gradually, it could easily become just another version of 'normal' – you sometimes didn't notice it as anything that odd. Perhaps, up till now, Sarah had, to her mind, *been* coping, and it had taken this crisis to show her she was not.

Much as I looked forward to meeting her, however, I had realised I was woefully ignorant when it came to having a clue about the specifics of her disease.

Mike likewise. 'Incredible, really,' he'd commented the night before, once we were in bed. 'Not to mention lucky.' He was right. There was no one in the family who'd had multiple sclerosis, and neither of us knew anyone who had either. 'I think the only person I know of who has had MS is that guy at work – d'you remember?' said Mike. 'The one they thought had a drink problem, and almost got sacked? Poor guy. I wonder what happened to him in the end.'

And so it went on. Though, once again, being in the dark was not a new situation for us. When Sophia had come to us with Addison's disease, we'd had to learn a lot of medical stuff in a very short time just to be sure her illness was kept under control. Were it not, we'd been warned, she could die. This, thankfully, was different. Physically, Abby was just fine. And Sarah wasn't our responsibility. But we still felt we needed to understand things a little better if we were going to help Abby through this stressful period. At the very least there was the central – and still unanswered – question about what was going to happen with Sarah long term.

In the end, I'd gone downstairs and got the laptop, so we could get a better picture of what we were dealing with. And having familiarised ourselves a little with the mechanics of the condition, we'd spent what turned out to be a dispiriting half-hour, reading about the many ways multiple sclerosis could disable a person. Not the most edifying kind of bedtime reading.

But there was no point in being negative. One thing our reading had surprisingly thrown up was a prevailing sense of optimism. Though some people had the disease very aggressively, others seemed to have a cycle of illness and remission, with a few lucky ones living long and mostly manageable lives. Perhaps all would be well after all.

Abby came home from school and just had time to run upstairs and change out of her uniform before it was time for me to drive her to the hospital. Sarah was a patient at the big general hospital in the next town to ours and it would be at least an hour's drive. Thankfully we'd be doing it just before the rush hour, and would have missed the worst of it by the time we travelled back. I'd packed some sandwiches and a drink for Abby and brought my usual pile of gossip magazines. Apart from pleasantries, my role was essentially one of chauffeur. Supporter too, of course, but beyond that, this was all about them. It was completely new territory for me, this situation – a very unusual circumstance – and I'd already asked how I should play it. Both John and Bridget had told me that I had to take a back seat, and unless Sarah wanted to ask me anything about Abigail's day-to-day routine, then I shouldn't get involved, because one fact still applied: this child was in care now, and all decisions about her welfare were the responsibility of social services.

'So, all excited?' I asked Abby now, once we were in the car and under way. She'd changed into some jeans and a T-shirt and was carrying her *Glee* backpack. I'd suggested she bring the scrapbook we'd made together so she could show her mum what she'd written and the pictures she'd drawn. I saw her face form a look of enquiry now.

A look of hopeful enquiry, too. I cursed my choice of words. 'Oh!' she answered, her eyes widening. 'Is Mummy coming home tonight now?'

'Sorry, sweetheart. No, I'm afraid not. Not yet. I just meant were you excited about *seeing* Mummy. Bet you are, eh? And I bet she can't *wait* to see you.'

Despite my knowing Abby knew that this wasn't going to happen, it was sad to see her looking so crestfallen. She fell silent and began to chew the skin around her fingers, staring out of the window at the leaden February sky.

'There's a sandwich in the box there, I said. 'And a banana, if you'd like it. And a carton of juice. I think it's –'

'Will they have given Mummy tea yet, d'you think?' she interrupted. I watched her tap her watch face for about the fifth time since we'd got into the car. Perhaps the hands stuck sometimes.

I looked at the clock on the dashboard. 'Not yet, I think, no. It's still a bit early, so –'

'But it's teatime,' she said plaintively. 'If she doesn't have her tea now, they'll be all behind with her bath. And it's *Coronation Street* tonight.' She frowned, and then seemed to think of something else to worry her. 'D'you think they even *know* what days are Mummy's bath days?'

'Love, I'm sure Mummy will have told them. Anyway, it's a hospital and in hospital they tend to give you a bed bath *every* day.'

'What's a bed bath?'

'It's what they do when you can't get out of bed.'

This seemed to horrify her. 'Don't they *help* her?'

'Yes, I'm sure they do. When she needs to get up, of course they do. They –'

'I think I should write a list for them,' she decided, unclipping her seat belt.

'Sweetheart, don't undo that –'

'But I have to get some paper, so I can do a list for them. I've got some in my backpack. It won't take a second.'

'Love, please do up your seat belt. It's against the law not to wear your seat belt …'

But needless to say, by the time I had said this, she'd made a grab for her backpack and was already buck-led up again. 'I think I *must*,' she said firmly, rootling for a pen.

I let her sit and write for a few minutes, conscious that she was right – she probably did need to, if only to transfer her anxieties to the page.

'All done?' I asked, once it seemed she'd run out of things to add to it.

She seemed happier now. 'I think so. I've had to leave some of the food things. Do they have a list for the whole week on that menu card you told me about?'

I tried to dredge up a memory of when I'd last seen one. It had been a very long time back. 'I don't think so,' I said. 'I think it's a new one for each day.'

'That's a bit silly,' she said. 'It would be much easier if they did it for the week, wouldn't it? Then they'd know what to buy. Much more organised.' She began scribbling something else.

I could have given her five minutes' worth of hospital catering arrangements, and how patients came and went and how it wouldn't be practical, but as I didn't think it would calm her down any I decided against it.

'Speaking of being organised,' I said instead. 'It's going to be half-term in a week or so. Is there anything special you'd like to do? Any outings we could go on? Anyone from school you might like to have round to play? Or come and see a film with us, perhaps? I'm sure there'll be lots of things on.'

Abby shook her head, making her bunches dance around. Her list complete, she was back absently chewing on her fingers. I wondered about drawing her attention to the fact, but decided against. 'Hmm?' I urged. 'What d'you think?'

'I'm not sure we should arrange anything,' she said, having given the matter her usual moment of thought. I had never seen a child so young be so measured in what she said. 'If you don't mind, that is,' she added. 'What if Mummy's home?' I was about to answer, but before I could formulate the most diplomatic reply she answered herself anyway. 'And if she's not, we'll be going to visit her anyway, won't we?'

Which seemed to be the end of the matter for her. 'Of course we will,' I said. 'But that won't be all day *every* day, will it? I'm sure we can find *one* day to go out for a little treat. Maybe bowling. There's a thought. My Kieron loves bowling. You'll meet him soon ... Yes, there's a thought. Have you ever been bowling? For a friend's birthday or something, maybe?'

I was fishing, but she didn't seem to notice. She took her fingers from her mouth and shook her head again dismissively. 'I don't really have time to go out to birthdays.' She said the word birthday with a slight but discernible air of contempt.

'What, never?'

She shook her head again. But then her expression changed. 'I could, if I wanted. I do get invited. But I don't go. Everyone's always so silly ...'

'Silly? How?'

'Just ...' She sighed heavily. 'Just so *childish*.'

'But that's okay, isn't it? You know. When it's a party, and you're playing games and stuff?'

Abby frowned again. 'I mean just silly *all* the time. I mean the girls are. They just do silly things and talk about silly things. And *boys* ... And I just never understand why they find it all so *interesting* ...'

Again, the word 'interesting' held that slight note of irritation, as if she found herself beached on the shores of a foreign country, and couldn't seem to get her head around the crazy things the locals did. Which perhaps she couldn't. And perhaps wouldn't, given the few things she'd told me. Did she ever – *had* she ever – done any normal kids' things?

But Abby was spared the pain of any further Casey inter-rogations as the hospital buildings rose into a grey and brick bulk on the horizon and I became preoccupied, out of necessity, as I'd fully expected to, by the business of working out how and where to legally park the car. It wasn't a hospital I knew well, but at least it had the usual array of enormous signs, all groaning under the weight of so much necessary information: outpatients, main hospital, accident and emergency, nurses' accommodation, staff car park, X-ray, chapel, catering services and so on. Plus the reliably unhelpful list of named buildings, all given their titles in homage, no doubt, to various esteemed, long-dead medical notables. I scanned the visual overload and eventually found 'visitor parking', which, as I'd also expected, was about half a mile distant and, while bristling with warnings about the consequences of illegal parking, pretty thin on available parking spaces.

We found one in the end, however, after a short bout of anxious circling, and I had just enough coins for the pay and display. I said as much to Abby, as I rummaged in my purse. 'Next time,' I said, almost as a mental note to self, 'we must remember to bring enough change with us.'

I heard the zip on the backpack being opened once again. 'I'll make a new list for that,' Abby reassured me.

* * *

I'm not sure what I had expected. Our stint of internet research had thrown up so many images, both mental and visual, that I realised I had no ready picture in my mind for Sarah, just a general expectation that she'd in some way 'look' ill.

But she didn't. Yes, she looked as if some movements were causing her pain – I noticed her wince as she waved a hand to greet us, for example – but if you gave her a cursory glance, you'd never think her 'ill'. The only evidence that there was something serious going on – though I didn't know what – was that there was a mound under the blanket, where her legs were, which I presumed was the outline of some sort of cage or box, keeping the covers from touching her.

The ward the duty nurse had directed us to was a six-bedder, the last of several identical bays. There was only one other bed occupied in her section at present, it seemed: a sleeping middle-aged woman, the top of whose bedside cabinet was crammed with cards and flowers. It made the lack of either on Abby's mum's bed feel very stark and I cursed myself for not thinking to bring some.

Sarah, who looked to be in her early thirties, was quite well built, which gave her a healthy sort of glow, though I noticed that her hair, which was a caramel to Abby's blonde, was lank and looked as though it hadn't been washed for a while. She had the same eyes as Abby, greyish green and deep set, and as we drew nearer I could see dark circles beneath them. I tried to imagine what it must be like to be her – to be so ill that you were separated from your only child in this fashion. And worse, to know she was being cared for by strangers. How did that *feel*? I really couldn't imagine.

I put a broad smile on my face, conscious of her silent inspection. That at least wouldn't set any alarm bells ringing, I didn't think. Though I knew how to discipline children of any age and size (it had been my job for so many years now that I had long since perfected 'the look') I was not an intimidating-looking character. At just five foot nothing, and in sweatshirt and leggings, plus comfy boots, mine was not the kind of look that would alarm anyone. And though I had more that once been called an 'old witch' (due to my black hair – teenagers could be so imaginative) by the odd miscreant who'd fallen foul of me in my days working at the local comprehensive, where adults were concerned my problem was more usually of being *under*estimated.

'Nice to meet you,' I said, beginning to extend a hand but, unsure if she'd want to shake it, transferred it to the pocket in my jumper instead. I knew from our recent research that MS sufferers could have pain in their hands. I looked at the cage again. And their legs too, I guessed.

Abby had seen it too.

'Mummy, what's that?' she asked, alarmed. 'Why have you got a house on your leg?'

'I broke my ankle, poppet,' she explained. 'When I fell. Didn't they tell you that?'

Abby shook her head. 'No, they didn't,' she said indignantly.

'Compound fracture, unfortunately,' Sarah said, now looking at me. 'Hence all this. Never rains but it pours, eh?'

By now Abby had sped straight to the other side of the bed and placed a quick peck on her mother's cheek. Now she grabbed her arm and began stroking it. It seemed an odd way to greet her – I'd have expected her to fling her arms around her. But then I realised that perhaps Sarah was in more pain than she was showing; the way Abby was so gentle and restrained in her movements made me wonder at a long-standing unspoken agreement that she had to be careful how she touched her, for fear of hurting her.

Abby seemed different – very matter-of-fact now she was with her mum, the two of them clearly slipping into long-established roles. While I exchanged pleasantries with Sarah – difficult to do in such circumstances but clearly something she was as keen to cling to as I was – Abby fussed around, plumping pillows and firing questions at her mother about when she'd been bed-bathed (she'd taken in what I'd said to her, clearly), what she'd eaten, whether she was all right for all her various medications, how she'd been sleeping and whether she had enough clothes. The notes she'd made in the car were ticked off as she did this, and I couldn't help notice how clipped and precise her manner had become. It really was as if she'd morphed into a mini-professional carer. And, even more tellingly, how comfortable her mother seemed with this. I kept expecting Sarah to make her first enquiry about Abby's day, but Abby had hardly paused to draw breath and, once again, Sarah seemed happy to let her continue.

'Anyway,' I finished, conscious that this was precious time for them to be together, 'I'm going to go and grab myself a coffee and leave you two to it.'

This seemed to galvanise Sarah. 'Poppet,' she said to Abby, who was now busy rootling in the bedside cabinet for a comb. 'Up at the end of the ward – ask the nurse; she'll direct you – there's a little library of books. Do you want to choose one for us to read?'

Abby popped her head up, and nodded. 'What kind?' she asked.

'Oh, you choose,' said Sarah. 'You know what we like.'

Abby nodded again, and trotted back down the ward.

Sarah turned to me. She had clearly been anxious that we speak alone. 'Look,' she said, as Abby disappeared from the bay, 'I know what you're probably thinking.'

'I'm not –' I began helplessly.

'How it *looks*,' she went on, as if I should have known. 'I know, because the social worker's told me. But you must understand –' She really emphasised the 'must'. She looked at me earnestly. 'That, well, it's not what it must look like. She's honestly fine. *Really*. I don't think they quite get it ...' She paused, and formed her mouth into a thin smile. 'There is no one. There is really *no one*. So I have *had* to be single minded. Do you understand?' Her eyes seemed to be willing me to say yes. Even though I wasn't sure quite what I was supposed to be understanding.

'I like to think I do ...' I began again. 'I obviously have no personal experience of your situation, but –'

'It was always just so important that I made her independent.'

'She's certainly that,' I agreed, wondering whether to say any more. 'Though –'

Sarah's eyes flashed and I sensed I was on tricky ground here. 'She's very capable,' I went on. 'I can see that. Though she does seem, well, a little over-anxious, understandably. Which is why they asked Mike and I ...'

'But that's exactly what I *mean*,' Sarah said. This conversation was becoming more confusing by the minute. If she had a point to make, it was a long time coming. 'I've *had* to make her that way, for just this eventuality,' she said. 'I've relapsed before.' She sighed heavily. 'And once I'm over this, I don't doubt, at some point, that I'll relapse again. This is a bitch of a disease. You never know when it's going to get you. And it's always been my number one priority to be sure Abby can look after herself.' She paused, and I could see she was becoming upset now. 'The absolute last thing I ever wanted was to be a burden to Abby. It's just us, you see ...' The wry smile flashed back. 'Me and her against the world. What with her having no dad ...'

'He's not contactable at all?'

'No! No, not at all. Never been there. Not since before I even *had* her.'

'But maybe ...'

'Really, don't even go there. I told you. There's no one.' She looked past me, and then changed her expression completely. 'Ah, poppet!' she said brightly. 'What have you found? So.' She turned to me again. 'How long do we have, Casey?'

I turned around, to see Abby trotting up, clutching two big hardbacks. Chick-lit, by the looks of things. Obviously large print. Both pink. I checked the time on my mobile. 'Say, forty-five minutes? Would that be okay?'

'That'll be *perfect*,' Sarah gushed. 'Abby is *such* a brilliant reader, aren't you, poppet? Top of the class last term, weren't you?'

Abby nodded happily, pulling the visitor chair round, ready to commence her reading. Happily, but with that same air of brittleness. As if inhabiting a role.

I left them to it and had the nurse direct me to the restaurant, a little puzzled by my short exchange with Sarah. She'd seemed so anxious to get through to me, but I wasn't quite sure what to make of it. One thing was clear, though. I felt she'd been misguided. From what little I'd seen so far – and, admittedly, it hadn't been much – her determination not to be a burden on her daughter had been misplaced. In having Abby so independent that she could do everything for the pair of them hadn't she actually created the situation she'd been so anxious to avoid? She had actually made herself a burden, both physically and emotionally. With Abby feeling it was her responsibility to be her mother's sole carer, taking that responsibility away – as had now, in fact, happened – had left the poor child in a horrible, lonely limbo.

Surely the thing to have done was to get every scrap of care that was available so that Abby could at least have a shot at a normal childhood? A chance to do all the normal childhood things? As it was, she was now a fish out of water socially, with no support network of friends to help her through. Let alone loved ones.

What a grim thing, to have absolutely no family. And once again, I simply couldn't quite imagine how that felt. But I berated myself as I queued for my coffee. It was none of my business. I was simply there to foster Abby, and do the best job I could in terms of minimising her emotional fall-out. Sorting everything else in their lives out was the remit of Sarah and Abby's social workers, one of whom – from what Sarah had hinted anyway – had been busy trying to do just that. She clearly felt defensive about what had been said to her. But what *was* that? I felt an itch start – and itch that wanted scratching.

No, I told myself. Casey, just *leave* it.

Chapter 6

Despite my resolution not to get involved in things that weren't my business, Abby *was* my business and, if it concerned her, it concerned me. So I woke early on Friday morning in a determined mood and with a mental list of questions that needed answers. All of which meant that I couldn't get back to sleep, so by the time the alarm was due to go off I was already down in the kitchen, pen in one hand, a mug of strong coffee clutched in the other. Since I'd given up smoking, it was my only remaining vice, and one I wouldn't be giving up any time soon. I sipped the bitter nectar gratefully as I transferred the questions that had been teeming in my brain to a piece of paper. As soon as the taxi came and picked Abby up for school, I knew I had a couple of calls to make.

'Is it Christmas again?' asked Mike, trudging blearily into the kitchen and blinking in the brightness of the strip light. 'Seeing you up at this hour is giving me the strangest feeling of déjà vu.'

It was still pitch-dark, not even seven, and I'd already been up half an hour. I grinned at him. 'Love, if this were Christmas the turkey would already be in the oven, I'd have Slade blaring out, the Quality Street open, and by now I'd have pulled at least one cracker.'

I pushed my chair back and went across to make him a coffee too – a posh one, from the swish machine we'd treated ourselves to for Christmas. And speaking of Christmas, it was a fair observation. I was nuts about it, and would throw myself into it wholeheartedly, but for the rest of the year Mike was the early riser in the household, bringing the coffee up to me, not vice versa. 'Well, that's a relief,' he said, stretching and yawning. 'For a minute there I thought you'd be having me up in the loft looking for fairy lights.'

I passed him his coffee. 'Just couldn't sleep, that's all,' I told him. 'You know what it's like when you wake up and straight away your brain reminds you about all the things you need to do? So I thought I'd take a leaf out of Abby's book and make a list.'

Mike frowned as he sipped his drink. 'You're not stressed, are you love?' he asked, nodding towards the ceiling. 'About Abby? I mean, compared to Spencer … in fact, compared to *all* the other kids we've had …'

'No, not at all,' I reassured him, shaking my head. 'I'm just on a mission to find out what's going on there. You know, the more I know about this the harder it is for me to understand how the two of them could have become so isolated. You'd have thought *someone* would have known what was happening at home, wouldn't you? What about the GP? I mean, he or she must be prescribing drugs for her, mustn't they? Or the neighbours? Or, come to that, Abby's school. Surely they'd have noticed something? It almost beggars belief.'

Mike rolled his eyes. 'Love, you're asking *me* that? You're asking *yourself* that? Look at Ashton and Olivia. There's your answer, right there. Just remember the sort of things that went on in *that* household. Compared to that, let's be honest, this is *nothing*.'

Mike was right, of course. The siblings he'd mentioned – both now thriving in new permanent foster-families, thankfully – had come to us looking like a pair of Dickensian urchins: underweight, covered in scabs, eye-poppingly filthy and feral, yet still living with their parents in the sort of conditions that would have the RSPCA throwing their hands up in horror, let alone the NSPCC. And that was before you took the sexual abuse into account ... No, in comparison, this wasn't a big social scandal. Just a woman who, for whatever reason – blind optimism, maybe? – had seemed to have turned 'muddling through without troubling the outside world' into something of an art form.

This was confirmed when I rang Abby's school, after she'd left for it in the taxi, in the hopes that I'd be able to have a few words with her teacher. Knowing how school timetables tended to work was always a bonus, and I was spot on in being able to grab five minutes with the man, who was a youngish-sounding teacher called Mr Elliot.

'I'm completely gobsmacked,' he admitted, when I introduced myself to him. He had no idea that Abby had even been taken into care.

'I mean, I knew her mum had had to go into hospital,' he said. 'But nothing about her going to stay with a foster family or anything. I just assumed she was with other family members. Is this long term?'

I told him I didn't know. 'So no one's been in touch?' I asked, confused myself now about how this fairly important information had failed to get to him. Not that it didn't happen from time to time. It had only been a few days, after all, and perhaps Bridget hadn't yet got around to it.

'Not to my knowledge,' he said. 'Though that doesn't mean they haven't. The head teacher was away on a course all day yesterday, so it's possible that the news just hasn't trickled through yet ... This is a big school, and I wasn't in myself on Tuesday. These things happen, I suppose ... Anyway, thanks for letting me know now.'

'I'm sure social services will be in touch with you as well,' I reassured him. 'Oh, and just so you know, she'll be coming by taxi each day for the time being, and picked up by taxi as well. I was just phoning myself so we could have a chat about Abby. Under the circumstances, she has a number of issues, as you can imagine ...'

'Circumstances? Forgive me, but as I say, I'm not up to speed.'

'As a result of her mother's MS,' I began.

'Really? She's been diagnosed with MS? The poor woman.'

'Yes, but not recently,' I explained, once again shocked. He didn't *know* this? 'She's been suffering with it for years,' I went on. 'Abby's been her carer since she was little, apparently.'

Mr Elliot was even more stunned by this information and maintained he had absolutely no idea. So I spent a few minutes describing the situation, and filling him in on what had been going on at home – as described to me by John and Bridget – after which Mr Elliot seemed flabbergasted.

Not to mention embarrassed. 'I don't think anyone here knew anything about this,' he confirmed. And I believed him. He didn't sound like he was just covering his back. 'And you know, Mrs Watson, it explains a great deal. The lateness, the tiredness, the days she's come in missing kit or uniform …'

So they had noticed *something*. 'So why didn't the school get in touch with her mum?' I asked him.

'Oh, believe me, we have. I can think of at least half a dozen letters that have gone home – by post, this is. Not to mention countless phone calls as well. But you know, there's always been a response from Abby's mum. And with a plausible excuse as to why, as well. We just – well, I hesitate to say it to you now – but we just thought she was a slightly introverted, slightly difficult child. Only child, of course, and sometimes they can have their own challenges, can't they? You know – with sharing and so on – connecting with their peers. Oh dear …' he tailed off. 'Oh dear, oh dear.'

I wasn't about to engage in a debate about only children. I'd dealt with children from all sizes of family in my past career, and if I knew one thing it was that you couldn't make blanket judgements about why children were the way they were. Some only children thrived, some kids from big families didn't. But, to be fair to Mr Elliot, he was somewhat on the spot, and probably feeling awful about not picking up on all this before.

'I know,' I said, 'but I can see how it happened. And you'll have only had her in your class for a term and a bit, anyway, wouldn't you?' He agreed he had. 'And from what I've seen so far, I think her mum's been very keen to be self-supporting. It's just that perhaps she was being unrealistic about just how sick she was. The collapse has at least brought things out into the open. Perhaps now she'll get some proper help and support. Anyway,' I finished, 'I'm glad I've been able to put you in the picture. Let's hope that between us we can help Abby through all this. School's an important routine right now for her, of course, and she does have a need to keep to routines. Just one last thing –'

'Of course,' Mr Elliot answered.

'Friends. Abby's adamant she doesn't actually have any. Is she really that isolated from her peers? Only she has her birthday coming up and I wanted to arrange something for her, but without some friends to invite I don't know if it's even feasible.'

I heard a sigh. 'I'm afraid she's telling you the truth,' Mr Elliot said sadly. 'I mean she mixes okay in class – well, up to a point – as best as can be expected. But, well, between you and me, she has something of a temper. Very easily irritated. She does tend to turn other kids off. I've not had a parents' evening with her mother yet, to be honest. But it would definitely be something I'd be mentioning to her. It's not that she's bullied or anything. Just that, well, as I say, she doesn't seem to *want* friends. She really is a loner, I'm afraid.'

And now I knew that Sarah always had answers to the school's concerns, I could see how easy it had been for Abby to remain under the radar.

Schools were busy places, and this one was a large one. And there were likely to be all too many kids constantly *above* the radar and causing a whole lot more grief.

Kids like the ones I generally fostered myself.

I called John afterwards, both to update him on things generally and to fill him in on school and pass on the message that Abby's teacher had been completely in the dark. And then I put the whole thing out of my mind and decided to get on with my day. After all, my role in all this was simply to take care of Abby for as long as was needed – not concern myself with whatever was going on with her mother. Of course I couldn't know then just how dramatic the consequences of 'concerning myself with Sarah' would be.

But for now, it was just a small itch of curiosity, easily put out of sight and out of mind. I did my housework with my mind on my own family, mostly, happy that Riley would be over with the little ones the following day. I adored my grandsons as much as any self-respecting nanna, and time spent with them was always very precious.

It would also, I thought, be nice for Abby to meet them, and something of a distraction for a little girl who had way too much of the weight of the world on her shoulders and not a soul – from what Mr Elliot had said – to support her. That she was feeling it was growing ever more obvious as well. When Abby arrived home from school I'd intended to sit her down and see if we could make a little progress with that, at least in relation to school. Once John had fed my news through to Bridget, and she'd been in touch with them herself, perhaps they could start taking measures to keep a closer eye on her and help her through this difficult period.

I made some pancakes, which I could microwave for when she got in, and pondered this odd little girl. Because she'd come to us so suddenly we still hadn't really had a chance to get to know all her likes and dislikes. As this obviously hadn't happened, filling it in with Abby now might be the perfect way to get her to open up a little about herself and give me an opportunity to probe a little deeper into school and friendships.

But I was unprepared for how strung out she clearly was. She'd come in from school pale and drawn-looking, and with half her packed lunch uneaten. And though she accepted a hot chocolate, she refused anything else, adamant that she wasn't hungry. I didn't press it. I had a feeling it would just stress her more, and at a time when she had more than enough to contend with. And not just with her mother – though she was co-operative enough about answering my questions (even a little animated describing the things she most enjoyed on TV, however unusually adult her choices), as soon as I mentioned having spoken to her teacher her eyes immediately filled with tears.

'It's all right, sweetie. You're not in any trouble,' I reassured her. 'I just needed to have a chat with Mr Elliot this morning, so he knows who I am and that you're staying here, that's all.'

'But I couldn't help it!' she spluttered, as if she wasn't even taking in what I was saying, the tears now spilling onto her cheeks. 'I couldn't!'

I felt mortified. The last thing I wanted was to upset her. But upset her I clearly had. She was looking really distressed. 'Couldn't help what?' I asked her gently, getting up from the kitchen table and returning with some tissues. 'Sweetheart, you're not in trouble, I promise,' I said. 'What is it? *What* couldn't you help?'

'About the rota for the *beans*! And I said I was sorry!'

I had no idea what she was talking about, and gently said so. Upon which she explained, juddering, through both tissue and tears now, that she'd been supposed to be the one watering some bean seeds her group had been growing for an experiment, and how she'd come into school late and forgotten and she'd *already* been told off, but how someone's bean had died now and they were all saying it was *her* fault and someone had been really nasty and called her names and how everybody hated her. And so on. This had been on Monday – so before everything had happened with

70

her mum – but the girl, who was apparently called Hayley (I made a mental note: not one for the party list, then), had got everyone to gang up on her and how it was just *horrible*.

'But I couldn't help it!' she said again, distress morphing into indignation. 'I have to go to the post office on Monday!' she sobbed. 'To get mummy's money. And they don't open till nearly school time and if there's a queue I have to wait!'

'You do this every week?' I asked her.

She looked surprised at the question. 'Of course,' she said. 'Monday is money day. If I didn't, we wouldn't have anything to eat, would we?'

Which was a valid enough point. And there was no point in my asking if the teachers knew about this, because I already knew the answer to that one.

'And I just get so *tired*,' she said, her shoulders slumping. She began turning the half-empty chocolate mug around in her hands. Round and round it went, in slow, precise circles. 'That's why I forget things,' she explained. 'I didn't mean to forget. I just get so tired when I'm in school.'

'I'm not surprised,' I said. 'What with all the things you do for Mummy. I'd be tired too. *And* forgetful. But that's one of the reasons I needed to speak to Mr Elliot,' I added slowly, keeping an eye on her expression, in case something I said unleashed another flood. 'Because if they know, they can help you better, and make sure the other children –'

'How can *they* help me?' she wanted to know. 'I shouldn't be made to *go* to school, even. Least, not that much. I have too many more important things to do at home. And what if Mummy falls over? She falls over and she can't get back up again. What if *that* happens when I'm at school? An' she can't get to the toilet, or anything?'

There was something about the way she said this that made me prick up my ears. '*Has* that happened, Abby?'

I could see her chin dimpling and her eyes filling up again. She didn't answer. Which I took to mean yes. On *both* counts. What an image. How on earth did she deal with something like that? She was so slight, for one thing, so, physically, it would be a struggle. And what about psychologically? And there being no one to tell. No one to share it with. How could any mother consider that an acceptable state of affairs? I got out of my seat and squatted down beside Abby's. Unlike many of the kids I dealt with, she didn't seem to have any attachment issues, at least; as before, she seemed happy enough to let me pull her into my arms. I could feel her sobs against my chest. 'I just want Mummy back,' she mumbled brokenly into my sweatshirt. 'I just want my *mummy* back. I want to go *home*. *Please*. When can I *go HOME*?'

'I know, my love.' I said, rubbing her back and hugging her. 'I know.'

I just didn't know when I could give her an answer.

Chapter 7

'Listen, winter,' declared Riley, peering miserably out of the kitchen window. 'We've had enough of you now. Go AWAY!'

It was Saturday lunchtime and the rain was coming down in stair rods, bouncing off the garden furniture that sat huddled on the patio, and turning the whole of our pretty new back garden into a bog. Right now there was such a big pond on the sagging trampoline that I wouldn't have been surprised to find ducks sitting on it. Not to mention frogspawn and a pair of koi carp.

I didn't mind the rain myself – it was what made Britain so green and pleasant, after all – but if there were two things that were often incompatible as bedfellows it was rain and stressed mothers with under-fives to keep entertained.

'It'll stop,' I reassured my scowling daughter, as I joined her at the window. 'You wait. Look. That's a patch of blue up there, isn't it?'

Riley snorted. 'Mother, what are you like? *Blue?* Come on – that's just a very slightly different shade of grey. Even your positive mental attitude doesn't have the power to change that.' She turned around. 'So, what shall we do then? Play shops? Make some fairy cakes? Take to the bottle ...?'

'Er, go down to the woods?'

'What, as in *swim* there?'

We might have moved house, amassed two grandsons and taken on a new foster child, but some things in the Watson family never changed. Riley and I tended to spend our Saturdays together, while Mike and Kieron did their weekly bit of father–son bonding. Of all the routines Kieron loved (and he loved his routines) having his dad watch him play Saturday league football was his favourite. If Mike wasn't on the touchline it would thoroughly spoil his day. So, come rain, shine or hurricane, Mike would always be there.

Though one thing, it occurred to me, had changed. Now Kieron was living with his girlfriend Lauren, in a self-contained flat above her parents, I was at least spared the Herculean task – and it would be Herculean, on a day like this – of trying to get the mud out of my son's kit. And we'd half-planned, Riley and I, to take the little ones on an adventure. It had been such a whirlwind moving into the house, and what with Christmas and New Year, there'd been little opportunity explore the place yet. And it was an area I hardly knew, so I'd been itching to get out and about to investigate our surroundings properly. I'd also spotted that there was a footpath off the green in front of the house, which the lady in the shop had said led down to a little patch of woodland. Perfect for little ones, she'd said (I'd been in there at the time with Levi), as it even had a little stream, where we could go pond dipping.

I'd also fancied getting out because I thought it would be good for Abby. The weekend had started badly, with the early morning news from John Fulshaw that Sarah had contracted some sort of viral infection. We had planned to go and visit her again early evening, but this was now out of the question, both because she was too poorly, and because of the risk of spreading the infection. John could only pass on the news that they'd update us on Sunday.

With her mum already so unwell, I knew Abby would be really traumatised about the news and I'd dreaded having to tell her. Once she'd got over her upset after school the previous evening, she'd talked of little else other than seeing her mum again, and making sure the hospital were looking after her properly.

She'd reacted as I'd expected, her eyes filling once again with tears, and I felt dreadful that I couldn't even promise her she'd see Sarah on the Sunday either, because, no matter how much I reassured her and plied her with that positive mental attitude of mine, I knew all too well the sort of thoughts that must have been going through her mind.

But I'd been right in thinking that my grandsons would prove a useful distraction. As soon as they arrived, it was as if the storm cloud over her own head had been spirited away. Within minutes of meeting them, she was completely besotted. Which, endearing as they were, I actually found fascinating initially. You could usually get a sense of how older children would be with little ones, and it was more often than not the case that the kids in big families were more at ease around babies. It stood to reason; children with lots of siblings, and perhaps nieces and nephews, just felt more relaxed around babies and toddlers because they were used to having them around. Only children, on the other hand, sometimes had difficulties relating. Without other children in their home lives they were often more used to solitude and their own space, and found the behaviour of little ones challenging. Snatching toys, creating chaos out of order, throwing tantrums – I'd seen it often. All behaviours that could make such children irritable.

It was a generalisation, of course, and a 'rule' that was often broken, but, given what we already knew of Abby, my hunch was that though she might enjoy playing with Levi and Jackson for a bit, she would soon find them a little bit tiresome. After all, she found the other kids in school difficult to deal with and, given her home life, she was clearly a solitary child.

Which was one of the reasons I'd been keen to get out on a long walk. Yet it had not been the case – far from it. Straight away she'd set about entertaining the pair of them, dragging out the toy boxes I kept in the hall, under the stairs, and suggesting games she could set up for the little ones to play. It was almost as if she was a mini playgroup leader, and the boys – even Jackson, who was still at that slightly clingy stage – were happy to let her organise them.

'She's a sweetie,' remarked Riley, who had returned from her vigil at the kitchen window and was now preparing some pasta for our lunch. We'd eat at home now, as opposed to going out with some sandwiches, as we'd originally planned, and see how the sky looked after that. If the worst came to the worst then we'd stay in and make those fairy cakes – why not? – but I was still hopeful we'd get out at some point.

I nodded, watching how Abby followed Jackson's every move, like a particularly over-anxious mother hawk. They were over on the other side of the dining room, building a castle out of Duplo, and all three were engrossed in the task. 'I feel so sorry for her,' I told Riley, keeping my voice low. 'I'm just so aghast how she's soldiered on so long without anyone having twigged to what was going on at home.'

I told Riley about the conversation I'd had with Abby's teacher, and about what John and Bridget had found at the house, and how isolated Abby had become. Riley shook her head. 'Unbelievable,' she said. 'What was her mother *thinking*?'

'That she'd be less of a burden on Abby, if Abby knew how to look after herself. That's what she told me, anyway.'

Riley's face made her feelings clear. 'Look after herself? Or her mother? Because that sounds more like it to me.'

'I'm sure there must be an element of that,' I agreed. 'But I don't think that was her intention. I think she really thought she was doing the right thing. I –'

I stopped then, as Abby was fussing around Jackson, who was trying to head off for a quick cruise around the coffee table but was being restrained, much to his annoyance, by her holding onto his dungaree straps. He was growing in confidence every day and he'd be walking soon, I reckoned. If he was allowed to, that was. 'He's fine, sweetie,' I reassured Abby, who was looking anxiously in our direction. 'Just let go of him. He'll be okay. And if he falls on his bottom, that's fine. It's all part of him learning ...' At which point, of course, Abby having grudgingly relinquished her hold on him, he did fall. And quite sharply, too, having been straining against her.

Abby's wail of anguish drowned out Jackson's one of frustration, and she scooped him up as if he'd toppled ten feet, rather than ten inches. 'Honestly, love,' Riley tried to reassure her also, 'he's fine!'

Abby wasn't mollified, and still cradled a by now wriggling and indignant Jackson. 'But he could have fallen against the coffee table and hit his head!' she persisted. She let him go, however, as he was getting ever more cross in her grasp. She stood up instead, looked around, and seemed to consider. 'Perhaps I should move the table, do you think?'

We both watched in amusement. She was already reaching for the pile of magazines and the TV remote that were on it.

'There's no need ...' I began. Then I thought better of stopping her. 'But if you'll feel happier, then by all means. You could slide it around behind the armchair.' I indicated where. 'Do you want me to come and help you?'

Silly question. Getting 'help' was an alien concept for Abby. The job was done before I could even finish speaking.

Matters didn't change much over lunch. I was beginning to realise that Abby was incapable of relaxing in the presence of the little ones. By the time we had finished preparing the food there had been major health and safety work accomplished in the living room. Presumably thinking I wouldn't mind, since I'd been happy enough about her moving the coffee table, Abby had set to work building a little fortress for the three of them. She'd removed all the seat and back cushions from both the sofa and the armchairs and the three of them were now playing Duplo in what looked like some sort of World War One foxhole.

I didn't mind at all, but once we called them all for lunch itself I began to get an unexpected insight into just how ingrained and acute her anxiety was.

'Is it okay if I feed Jackson?' she asked Riley politely, as we sat down.

'Of course you can, sweetheart,' Riley answered. 'If you want to. Be my guest.' Jackson didn't really need much help with eating these days, of course. He ate a lot of what we did, and loved feeding himself, too, so by now Riley would only feed him if we were eating on the hoof and she didn't want the usual attendant mess.

And he was happy enough to let Abby feed him, in any case; like all little ones, he enjoyed the attention. But Abby was much too stressed to enjoy it herself. 'I think this spaghetti needs mashing up, doesn't it?' she asked me anxiously. She was already busy crushing the strands to a virtual pulp. 'Or he might choke, mightn't he? You can't be too careful, you know.'

'It's just fine, love,' I reassured her. 'He can't choke on it. It's too soft.' Even so, she began giving him the tiniest little mouthfuls, and it was no wonder he kept trying to grab the spoon out of her hand.

Levi, seated the other side of her, was another cause for her hawk-eyed concern. 'Open wide,' she kept saying, every time he spooned up a new mouthful. 'I need to check your mouth's empty before you put any more food in.'

Levi, clearly bemused, would obediently do so, but after the sixth or seventh time of being inspected in this fashion he turned to me, confused. 'Nana,' he wanted to know, 'is Abby a little mummy?'

Which had us all smiling, Abby included. However, it didn't escape my notice – though again I didn't press it – that her own lunch was largely untouched.

We did get our walk in the end, though it ended up being the Sunday before we could head down to explore the woods, when the clouds had finally shifted enough for us to enjoy a little sunshine, even if it was boggy under foot. We'd had a second call from John, too; Sarah was okay, sent her love and would call Abby that evening, but they felt it inadvisable for her to visit that day. They hoped we'd be able to visit again on Monday or Tuesday, which news Abby took on board without too much visible upset.

But the constant tension that I realised seemed always to be around her soon began to manifest itself again. We headed out and the little patch of woodland turned out to be delightful. A tract of land that had been preserved between two large areas of housing, it followed the course of a stream that tumbled down a slight incline, and was criss-crossed with several meandering paths. It was obviously a haven for dog walkers and children, and even in gloomy February, with very little growing yet, it was, I decided, a real find.

But I wasn't sure Abby could even see it, let alone enjoy it. It was as if, in Levi and Jackson, she had found something else to get herself worked up about. It certainly seemed to be the only thing on her mind.

'So,' Mike had asked her, as we'd headed down the pathway across the green. 'Did you enjoy playing with Levi and Jackson yesterday?'

This simple enquiry had unleashed a kind of torrent; it was as if she'd spent the whole of the previous night worrying and now needed her fears about them to be allayed. Did Riley, she wanted to know, know how to look after them properly? Did she understand about filling a bath with cold water before hot water so there was no danger of scalding them accidentally? Did she understand about germs? Did she have a fire blanket and did she keep it somewhere accessible? Did she have stair gates that she kept closed at all times?

Mike chuckled as we began to make our way through the woods. 'Oh, don't you worry. Of course she does,' he reassured her, glancing across at me, his expression one of mild amusement. 'Fixed to the wall, they are,' he added. 'They even borrowed my drill to do it. And, actually, now I think about it, I'm still waiting for it back.'

'How d'you know about stair gates and all that stuff, love?' I asked her. I wondered if she had more experience of little ones than I'd first thought. And if so, from where? Maybe Sarah wasn't so isolated after all. Maybe there was a friend we didn't know about.

Abby carefully negotiated an expanse of muddy water before answering. This was clearly not a child who'd jump in a puddle. She would probably be thinking too much about the laundry it might create. 'From my book,' she said, as if surprised that I wouldn't already know that.

'What book's that, love?' asked Mike, doing likewise, in a single squelchy stride.

Abby watched him, edging back a little. I could swear I saw her wince. 'My safety book,' she answered. 'Don't you have one? Doesn't Riley?'

I shook my head. 'Safety book?'

Abby nodded. 'It's called *Look Out!* Mummy got it for me. I think she bought it off the internet. I've got three of them, actually. But Riley can borrow them. I don't mind. If someone can go and get them ...'

'That's really kind of you,' Mike said, 'but you keep it safe at home. Don't worry. Riley knows what to do. Here, look,' he said, pointing. 'Here's that stream Casey was on about.' He took a couple more steps, then squatted down on his haunches to scrutinise it more carefully. It was actually more like a stepped series of ponds. 'I'll bet there'll be tadpoles in there before too long. And a few stickleback. It's just the sort of –'

'But *does* she?' Abby's voice was a sudden plaintive squeak behind him. She obviously had no interest in pond-life. 'I bet she doesn't. Not everything. Do you *know* how many accidents happen in the home, Mike? Well, *do* you?'

We both stared at her, taken aback by this unexpected little outburst. And, as had kept happening, once again her eyes immediately filled with tears. I rushed to put my arms around her, but she stiffened at my touch.

'You shouldn't laugh! You just don't *realise*!' she spluttered, shrugging me away. 'The home's a very dangerous place!'

'Sweetheart, I know it *can* be,' I said gently. 'As I'm sure your book says. But, you know, you really mustn't worry about Levi and Jackson. Yes, accidents can happen. And, you're right – sometimes they do. But, you know, Riley and David *do* know how to take care of them. They're very careful. As I know you'll be if you have children of your own one day, too.'

Abby's eyes blazed at this. 'I'm not having any children! Ever! I just want mummy back! Why won't they let me have my mummy back? I *hate* them.' She turned to Mike. 'And I hate *you* as well!'

And with that she turned and ran away from us.

Chapter 8

Oh God, I thought, as Mike and I set off in pursuit. Please don't let us have another runaway. Spencer had really run us ragged in that regard – 'run' being the operative word. In the few months he'd been with us, he'd gone AWOL pretty constantly, more than once being missing overnight. He was a proper little Houdini, and incredibly street-wise for an eight-year-old, and in the end we'd had to keep the house locked up like a prison – including all the upstairs windows. He was such an old hand at absconding he had every angle covered – and that had even included making getaways by shimmying across roofs, like a character in a cartoon.

Thankfully, Abby, though impressively fleet of foot, hadn't figured on the perils of running over deceptively soft rain-sodden leaf litter. She'd headed off at quite a lick along the stream bank, but had barely covered a hundred yards before tripping on something – a buried log or tree root or tangle of brambles, probably – and going down hard into the cold peaty soil.

She was still face down when we got to her, her shoulders heaving as she sobbed, now as much in frustration, I didn't doubt, as distress. Mike was there first, and helped her up from the muddy ground, and I looked on in dismay at the state she was in. Her previously pale pink hoodie was now liberally streaked with chocolate-coloured mud, and you could hardly see the fabric of the front of her jeans. Worse, her hands and face were caked in it and as she held the former up to the latter she let out a wail that could have brought bears out of hibernation, had there been any in this neck of the woods.

'Sweetheart, don't cry,' I tried to soothe, as she looked at her palms in horror. You could see she didn't know quite what to do with them. There was no part of her she could rub them on that wasn't already covered. I had a packet of tissues in my jacket pocket, but it seemed pointless to even proffer them. It would be like trying to use a pedalo to cross the Atlantic. I cursed myself. I invariably went everywhere with wet wipes these days, as well as sanitising hand gel. It was one of those things that went with nanna territory. But not today. We were only popping out, the three of us, after all.

Thankfully Mike had his wits about him. 'Come on, Abby,' he said. 'Back to the bank, eh? Let's rinse those hands off, at least. Then we can get you home and in the bath, can't we, while Casey works her usual miracles with the washing machine. She's a veteran, you know. Muddy kit's her forte.'

Abby nodded mutely and stepped gingerly where Mike indicated, and I was glad I'd at least persuaded her to borrow a pair of wellies from the vast supply I had amassed over the years. The one pair of trainers she'd come to us with were almost impossibly clean and white, testimony to the sad fact that unlike most of her contemporaries she didn't spend her free time doing what other children did. But they would have been white no longer, had I allowed her to wear them. So that was something at least.

She was still sniffing back tears as we returned to the side of the stream, holding her hands out in front of her, horrified – almost as if they didn't even belong to her, but had been tacked on to the end of her arms against her will. 'Don't you worry,' I said, as Mike pointed out a place where there was water falling into a pool from a slight overhang. 'I'll have everything clean as new. Mike's right. If they gave out Oscars for getting stains out of stuff, I'd have had to build a bigger mantelpiece to display mine on, I'd have so many!'

But Abby was far too preoccupied with the mud all over her to really listen, and clearly not in the mood to be jollied along. So instead I shut up, squatted down beside her and Mike, and helped her by rolling her sleeves up. She'd obviously feel much happier once her hands were at least clean. Then we could set off and get her home and in the bath.

'That's the way,' said Mike, as she rubbed them together under the water. I dipped a finger of my own in. It was clear and ice cold to the touch. The mud sloughed off her palms easily enough, but also revealed a cut. She had a big scratch across the ball of her thumb, bless her.

'Ooh, you poor thing,' I soothed. 'I'll bet that's stinging now, isn't it?'

But Abby didn't answer. Once again she let out a wail of distress.

'Oh, sweetheart,' I said. 'I know. But we'll be home soon and we can get some cream on it. And a nice big fat plaster ...'

Now Abby looked up at me with huge tear-filled eyes. 'But we have to go to hospital,' she sobbed, 'or I'll die!'

This was, I reflected, as I gathered up Abby's discarded clothing, not only new but very confusing territory. You get used to things as a foster carer. And perhaps Mike and I, given the kind of extreme foster caring we usually did, had had the opportunity to get used to more than most. We had dealt with all kinds of self-harming, with being threatened with knives ourselves, with kids so badly neglected that they were feral and crawling with lice. We'd dealt with everything from inappropriate sexual behaviour in children barely out of nappies, to extreme violence and suicide attempts.

And that was just as foster carers; in my previous role as a behaviour manager I'd seen more damaged children in an average week – doing damage to both themselves and others – than some teachers in some schools might see in a whole term.

Abby was different. She was loved. She was cherished. She'd been wanted. Yet she was damaged too, and quite profoundly. She had been so upset by the cut on her hand that it took us till we were half the way home – Mike had scooped her up and carried her in the end – to manage to get out of her why she was so sure she was going to die.

Tetanus had been the answer. She was convinced she now had tetanus. And when she'd calmed down enough to speak she was quick to point out why. She'd been cut in the outdoors and that's 'where tetanus happened'. It lived underground and it didn't like the air. So you got it by being cut when you were out playing in the garden, because the germs went straight from under the ground to under your skin, so they didn't go in the air so they didn't die.

But you *did*. She seemed to know absolutely everything about it, no doubt from both her mum *and* one of her books. So it took us both a long time to reassure her that she didn't have to worry because it was only a scratch, and that tetanus was extremely rare, and was only a problem with deep outdoor injuries, such as standing on a rusty nail or something.

'Besides,' Mike had pointed out, as he pulled off her wellies, 'you'll have had an inoculation against tetanus when you were a baby, so even if you *had* had a nasty injury of that kind, the bug couldn't live in you anyway.'

'But if we don't get those clothes off and in the washing machine pronto,' I added, 'that mud will start feeling *way* too at home. Come on, missy, let's get you upstairs and in that bath, eh?'

Abby let me pull the hoodie over her head and took her socks off. She kept coming back to her hand – which to

calm her I had wrapped up in half a dozen of my tissues –
and still didn't look as if she was convinced.

'But what if I didn't?' she wanted to know, as we trooped
upstairs to the bathroom.

'What, have your immunisations? Oh, you'll have had
them, trust me. All babies do.'

'But what if Mummy didn't take me? What if she was
too poorly that day and missed it?'

'She won't have,' I said firmly. 'She absolutely won't
have. So. Bubble bath. I have vanilla or I have ... let me see
... Japanese garden. Which scent would madam prefer?'

'But that is a point, to be fair. She *might* have missed it,'
said Mike, once Abby was busy soaking in her cherry
blossoms. 'I mean, you don't know, do you? How would
we?'

'Oh, lord, don't you start,' I said, as I gratefully grabbed
the coffee he'd made for me. I was still feeling the cold and
could have done with a soak myself. I pulled out a kitchen
chair and sat down. 'Of course she'll have had her jabs.
God, you're going to get me all twitched now.'

'I'm just saying,' said Mike. 'We know hardly anything
about her, after all.'

'Well, it's something I can check easily enough, I guess.
I might have to register her with Doctor Shackleton in any
case. So I can ask him to check, can't I? But she *hasn't* got
tetanus. That was just a tiny scratch from a bramble, which
barely scratched the surface. I think I'd know if it was the
sort of wound that was deep enough for tetanus to be a

worry. And I'll put some Savlon on it anyway, and …' I looked at Mike. Who was grinning at me now. '*What*?'

He continued grinning. 'Just you,' he said. 'And for what it's worth, I agree with you. But she's a funny little thing, isn't she? I meant to mention earlier. Have you noticed that thing she does with her sleeve?'

'What thing?'

'I noticed it yesterday, and then again this morning. She always pulls her sleeve over her hand when she opens a door. Like this –' Mike pulled his jumper sleeve over his own hand to demonstrate. 'And one time yesterday, I noticed, when she didn't have a sleeve long enough, she spent about five minutes trying to do it with her elbow instead.'

'I hadn't,' I said. 'But it fits with everything else we know, doesn't it? The health and safety obsession and so on. The million times a day she seems to need to wash her hands. It definitely figures.'

'I was going to mention that too,' Mike said. 'Endlessly.'

I sighed. 'Poor little thing. I mean, I know in the grand scheme of things it's not so bad, really. I mean, not when you compare her to someone like Justin, at any rate. But even so.'

Justin had been our first foster child and I loved him dearly. We still saw him regularly – he'd never stop being part of our family – and if ever there was a child with the world on his shoulders, it had been him. The child of a drug-addicted mother, he'd been in care since he was five, when he'd burned down the family home.

How damaged did you have to be to do such a thing? We soon learned. He'd then spent the next few years bouncing back and forth between his feckless mother (who would pick him up and drop him with as much care as an inept knitter) and countless children's homes and foster homes. His eventual tally of 20 failed placements was a shocking number for a span of just five years – and he'd grown steadily more damaged with every move. By the time we got him, aged ten, he'd been given up on by just about everyone. No, compared with Justin, I reminded myself, Abby's problems weren't *that* bad.

Except, of course, they *were*. Or soon would be, if her life wasn't straightened out. It wouldn't take much for this traumatised child – missing her mother, adrift, anxious, friendless and bewildered – to become irretrievably psychologically disturbed. In some ways, I thought, social services had shown great prescience in addressing that fact, because her mother clearly hadn't.

And it was our job to try to stop that happening. I drained my cup of coffee in determined mood. 'But that's what we're here for, eh?' I said, as much to myself as to Mike. 'And look at the time. She's got to be clean by now, even by her exacting standards.'

'Even if her clothes aren't,' commented Mike, looking at the filthy heap on the kitchen floor.

Having scooped up the offending items and filled the bowl with water to soak them, I was just about to go up and see how Abby was doing when she reappeared. She looked pink and fresh again, and with an expression that was marginally brighter. Perhaps now she'd had a soak she could accept that the scratch on her hand was only minor. Or perhaps she was just resigned to whatever fate was in store.

She glanced at the bowl. 'I'm really sorry, Casey,' she said, her expression serious. 'I was being silly, running off like that, wasn't I?'

'Oh, no harm done,' I said lightly. 'It's been an upsetting time for you, sweetheart. We understand, really we do.' I was on my knees under the sink by now, pulling out my plastic box of heavy-duty laundry aids, and when I looked up I saw her wan smile turn to one of relief and pleasure. Well, that was what it seemed to be, at any rate. Even if I couldn't work out why.

She came across and joined me on the kitchen floor, looking almost joyful. 'Oh!' she said. 'I was wondering where you kept all this stuff!'

I might just as easily have pulled out a box of Barbie dolls or cupcakes. 'It's my magic box,' I told her. 'Full of all my lotions and potions.' I did a little witchy cackle. 'All eventualities covered. Though spells and hexes only by arrangement.'

I was pleased to see I'd conjured a big grin from even her. She peered into the box excitedly. 'Are you going to do some cleaning? Can I help you?'

'Well, I was just going to find some stain-removing powder, so I can soak your jeans and hoodie before I wash them.'

'But while you're doing that ...' She pointed towards my trigger bottle of bleach spray. 'I could do some polishing and stuff ...' she paused and then said shyly, 'to be helpful.'

'Oh, you don't want to be doing that on a Sunday ...' I started. 'And besides, I'm such a clean freak, you'll be hard-pushed to find anything *to* polish!' But then I thought of what Mike had said about her worrying about germs on the doorknobs. Perhaps it would help her to settle if she cleaned them herself. Yes, that might be a useful plan. 'Well,' I said, 'I guess if you really want to, I suppose ... yes, I don't see why not.'

The effect was electrifying. She plunged her hands into the box as efficiently as any professional contract cleaner and, rubber gloves popped back the right way out and quickly donned, had both spray and the correct cloth in hand in moments. And within no time, while I attacked the bowl of muddy clothing in the sink, she set about attacking all the knobs on the kitchen cupboards. I clearly wasn't the only one who found contentment in cleaning, then.

'You know,' I said, once I'd changed the soaking water and added my magic powder, 'Jackson's going to be one soon and we're planning to hold a little party for him. And Mike and I were wondering if you'd like it if we made it a joint one, for your tenth birthday, since it's coming up soon as well. Would you like that?'

The anxiety flashed in her eyes once again. 'I don't have birthday parties,' she said, almost as if admonishing me.

'It's too much for Mummy. We always just have a special tea.'

I nodded. 'I understand,' I said carefully. 'It must be hard, with Mummy's illness. But while you're here ... and since we're going to be throwing a party for Jackson anyway. Well, I just thought – why not ask a few friends from school along too?'

Again, I felt her tension. 'But I might not be here next month, might I? And besides,' she persisted, 'there's no one. No one I'd *want* to come, anyway. They're all just silly. I told you ...'

She had, too. I couldn't argue that point. And I wasn't about to contradict her about when she may or may not be able to go home again. Not right now. And once again I felt saddened at how all this had come about. You didn't tend to maintain friendships when you were the perpetual outsider. When you never invited any of your peers round to play. And though it wasn't a nice thought, and a part of me felt guilty for thinking it, it occurred to me that Sarah couldn't let her daughter have friends round for parties, even if Abby wanted to. If she had, it would obviously mean interacting with their parents, which might mean someone realising the conditions in which poor Abby lived. Which might have profound repercussions ...

I was just reassuring Abby that she was under absolutely no pressure to ask anyone round when a key turned in the front door to reveal Kieron, closely followed by an excited and dripping Bob. Bob had been the family dog for getting on for three years now – since the day Kieron just arrived with him, fresh from an animal sanctuary. Though he no longer lived with us – he'd gone with Kieron, to Lauren's – he was still very much part of our home. Which was presumably why he still had no compunction about doing his drying off by shaking his wet coat in the middle of my kitchen.

'Hey, Mr!' I tutted. 'Thanks for that! *NOT*.' I pulled my own rubber gloves off, the cleaning spell clearly now over. What with everything, I'd lost all track of the time, not to mention the fact that Kieron had already told me he'd be popping over. He'd promised to come and sort half a dozen huge boxes containing some of his collection of CDs and DVDs, which, with the house move being so last minute, still required his attention. It was a collection that had been acquired over his entire childhood, and it really needed pruning, the plan being to decide which to take to his and Lauren's, which should go to the local charity shop and which were worth trying to sell on eBay.

Kieron being Kieron, this would be no simple task. With his Asperger's, he was pathologically obsessed about order, so this would be no simple 'keep, donate or sell' half-hour job. Even assuming he'd be able to part with half of them – and there was only so much room for, not to mention sense in, storing them – they would first have to be re-catalogued to the minutest degree.

'Oh, no, you don't,' I said to Bob now, before he could add to his crimes by launching himself – and his filthy paws – over an already cringing Abby. 'You're out of bounds till you've had a proper rub down!' I scooped him up – I was still in my muddy jeans, so it didn't matter. 'And I tell you what,' I said to Abby. 'I think we can call it a day with cleaning, don't you?' I grinned at my son, as he shrugged off his jacket, a perfect plan hatching in my mind. To some extent, I realised, these two were peas in a pod. I grinned at Abby while Bob enthusiastically licked my face. 'I'm betting Kieron here would love the chance to recruit you.'

'What's that, Mum?' Kieron asked, hanging his coat over the newel post. 'All right, Abby?' he greeted her. She nodded shyly.

'Your big DVD sort-out,' I explained. 'Abby's a complete whizz at getting organised, aren't you, sweetie? So why don't the two of you crack on while I make us all some tea?'

Abby nodded again. As did Kieron, who was obviously happy to have the company. And as I watched them trot off upstairs, I reflected that, even though, as peas went, they were very differently sized ones, my random thought might just turn out to be the best one I'd had all day. Abby might not have friends at school, but she might just find one in Kieron.

Though quite how much of a friend he'd turn out to be, bless him, I was yet to see.

Chapter 9

'Good news,' I told Abby when she returned home from school the following day. 'Mummy's feeling well enough again for us to visit her.'

I'd taken the call from Bridget that lunchtime. Sarah was apparently recovering from her fever, and though she was still very poorly she was keen to see Abby.

Abby's response, however, was typically brisk. 'About flipping time!' she blustered, pulling off her backpack and yanking her arms from her blazer, before hanging the latter neatly over the newel post. 'About flipping time!'

To my delight, the DVD sort-out with Kieron had been a great success. Not only had they cleared all six storage boxes between them, but Kieron had also given Abby the pick of all the kids' films as a thank you for all her hard work.

'You should have seen her, Mum,' he'd told me before he'd set off for home. 'She was like the cat that got the cream – and all over a few ancient Disney films!'

It had made me think, that. What had been throwaway items, almost – many of Kieron's movie collection had been picked up at boot sales and charity shops in the first place – were obviously things this child had simply never had. With no family to buy her presents, and a sick, often house-bound mother, who was probably chronically short of cash, such luxuries as DVDs might have been in very short supply.

After Kieron had gone I'd dug out an old DVD player for her to use, and set up our old portable for her bedroom. And it was Kieron she mostly talked about on the way to the hospital now. How funny he was and how generous he was. She also mentioned something I hadn't been aware of at the time – she'd told him how she'd never been allowed to have a pet, and he'd said she could have a 'virtual one' instead. He'd taken a photo of her and Bob on his smart-phone, and had printed it out so she could stick it in her scrapbook and show it to her mum when she visited. Hearing that, I felt that warm glow you always get when a plan comes together. I was also naturally very touched by what he'd done.

But for all her apparent jollity, Abby lapsed into silence as the hospital buildings loomed into view. I couldn't blame her. As reminders of 'grim reality' went, this was it. It had been one of those dull, drizzly days that make you think the winter's never ending, and in the dusky pewter light the hospital looked as bleak as could be. It had also started raining pretty heavily.

'Don't forget the scrapbook, then,' I reminded her as we parked up in the usual far corner of the car park. I peered at the heavens, and wished for my son's attention to detail. No hat and no umbrella, despite my popping the latter on the hall windowsill ready. Though at least Abby had a hood, so we wouldn't get completely drenched.

I fed the pay and display machine with the usual cobbled-together assortment of loose change, and we hurried up to the hospital buildings, dodging puddles. But if I was glad to get inside and reunite mother and daughter for a bit, my hopes for a fond reunion were to be quickly dashed.

Sarah had been moved to a side room now, which was something of a blessing, because the first thing Abby did on seeing her was to march up to the bed, slam her hands against her hip bones and glare at her mother.

'How much longer are you going to keep this up, Mummy?' she shouted. 'When are you going to have a remission? WHEN?'

Shocked both by her tone and by the unexpected decibel level, I caught up with her and placed a hand on her shoulder. She shrugged it off angrily. 'Mummy! What's going to happen to the house? It's going to go to the dogs! It'll be dis*gust*ing! Come on! We need to GO HOME!'

Sarah's face, initially registering bafflement, began to crumple.

'Poppet, I'm so sorry ...' was all she managed to get out before collapsing into shoulder-heaving sobs. And even crying looked painful. My heart really went out to her. 'Abby, love …' I began, but by now Abby had burst into tears too, and, once again shaking off my comforting arm, launched herself onto the bed and flung herself across her mother's chest.

'Oh, poppet, I'm so sorry,' Sarah said again, tears streaming down her face as she hugged her daughter. 'Mummy doesn't want to be ill. I just can't help it! Oh, Abby, I miss you so much! I'm doing my best, I promise! Please don't cry. Please don't …'

Once again, I could see Sarah's obvious discomfort. And I was acutely aware of my own, for that matter. I shouldn't be here, I thought. I was pretty sure Sarah didn't want me there, either. I took a step back, and then another, and since they were oblivious to me anyway I mumbled something about getting a drink, and scuttled out.

I remembered the brace of vending machines that were stationed just down the main corridor, and headed gratefully for them. Clearly in macabre mood (possibly a side-effect of the gloomy weather) I tried to imagine what it must be like to know you were dying and that you would have to explain it to your distressed, soon-to-be-orphaned child. Sarah wasn't dying – I did know that – but even so it was still upsetting. She wanted to take care of her child, her child wanted to be with her, yet they were at this horrible impasse, kept apart from one another, with the spectre of being permanently separated ever present. And it seemed that at any moment I was about to find out just how very likely that was looking.

I'd just arrived at the coffee machine and pulled my purse out of my handbag, when I could hear someone approaching behind me.

'Hiya,' a female voice said. 'You just brought Abby up, right?'

I turned around to see a young woman walking towards me. She was perhaps in her mid-twenties, with a bright smile and an enormous patchwork bag. I wondered if she was perhaps Sarah's social worker. I nodded. 'Just giving them some time alone.'

'I'm Chelsea,' she added, plonking the bag down on the row of seats beside the machines, while I fed coins – my last few – into the slot. 'I'm Sarah's occupational therapist.' Ah, I thought. Not right, but nearly. 'Well, for the present, at least,' she added. 'You're Casey, right? The social worker mentioned you.' I nodded. 'Poor kid. Sarah was explaining things to me. You just can't imagine how bad it must be for them, can you? Being separated like this. Poor little thing,' she said again. I was about to answer – in the affirmative – when she laughed, and re-grouped her features. 'Doh! What am I *saying*? You're a foster carer!' She pulled her own purse from a pocket in the bag and started rummaging in it for coins also, then smiled up at me. 'I'll bet you've seen far worse in your line of work.'

I smiled back as pulled my plastic cup from the holder. The contents looked reliably undrinkable. 'I've seen my fair share, I guess,' I said. 'But you're still right. It's just so sad, all this, isn't it?'

Chelsea's face now formed a professional frown. 'You're telling me. Horrible, *horrible* disease.'

'So I'm learning,' I agreed, as she began feeding her own coins into the machine. 'I've been trying to gen up on it. It's all new territory. I've no personal experience of it myself.'

'Hurrah to that. I have an aunt who has been living with it since her teens. It's part of the reason I became an OT. And it's particularly grim in Sarah's case, of course, now it looks like she's moving to secondary progressive. Not the best news, all things considered. And God – *how* unlucky was that wretched fracture? But, yes, grim all round. Though, truth be known, looking at what I've seen of her history, maybe she's never really been in the relapsing–remitting group anyway. Perhaps she's actually had primary progressive from day one.'

I sipped my grey coffee-flavoured water and duly grimaced. 'Now you've lost me.'

Chelsea smiled apologetically. 'Sorry. I tend to do that.' She then explained about the various types of MS you could have, and how one could morph into another – and often did – while another was benign ('Would that every kind were that kind, eh?'), and a fourth – and what it seemed they thought Sarah might have, which was increasingly disabling from the outset, with each relapse causing irreparable damage.

'So that's the one they call primary progressive – for obvious reasons. And it would seem to fit. This is certainly proving to be quite a severe relapse, isn't it? And, of course, given the home situation, it's *all* a bit grim, isn't it? Always difficult when patients have no one to support them at home, obviously. I mean, here by the grace of God and all that – where the hell do they *go*?'

'Exactly,' I said, because I'd wondered that myself. 'Where *do* they go?'

Chelsea sipped her own drink. 'God! How do they make this stuff so spectacularly grisly? What, you mean, in the short term? Well, off an acute medical ward, for starters, otherwise there'd be no beds left free for anyone. To nursing homes, often, to shuffle around with all the octogenarians. Can you *imagine*? But if they fulfil the criteria, or have the means to finance it, ideally to a dedicated rehab facility.'

I tried to imagine being in your thirties and having to move to a nursing home. Or a rehab facility, for that matter, though the latter sounded marginally better. 'What, as a live-in patient?'

She nodded. 'For a period of weeks, usually. Occupational therapy, physio, nutrition, the whole rehabilitation package. Till they can cope again independently, if that's possible, of course. With a lot of MS relapses, there's a critical period when they have a decent chance of regaining some function – miss that and you're scuppered, basically. Though in Sarah's case they're still thinking about that clinical trial first, aren't they? Which'll mean keeping her here for at least the next couple of weeks – they need close monitoring, of course. The drugs are pretty heavy duty.'

I shook my head. 'I don't know,' I said, growing anxious now about how much she was telling me, and realising that she thought I was privy to a lot more than I was. 'All I know is that I've got Abby for as long as she needs to be with me.' I frowned. 'Which from what you say is looking like it might be for a little longer than originally thought.'

I could see Chelsea's face turning a definite shade of crimson. 'Oh, God,' she said. 'I thought … I mean, I hope I haven't been indiscreet here. I assumed you knew about all this.'

'Not a great deal,' I admitted. 'As a foster carer you don't usually have very much contact with the birth family, for obvious reasons. Certainly nothing like this. It's an unusual case for us. But don't worry. I'm not in the habit of blabbing. And, trust me, the last thing I want is for Abby to know all this. Right now she's waiting patiently for her mum to get better. Thinking she's going to is what's keeping her going. As and when that changes – well, we'll have to cross that bridge when we come to it.'

'God,' Chelsea said with feeling. 'That poor mite.'

For all that it wasn't my business, I brooded about what Chelsea had told me all the way home. Having got her outburst out of the way, Abby seemed in better spirits. Well, if not in particularly good spirits, exactly, at least she seemed calmer for having vented her frustration at her mum, so perhaps it was all to the good that she'd got it out of her system. She badly needed an outlet for her doubtless myriad emotions, and, with no family or friends to draw on, she sadly lacked one.

But knowing what I now knew, I felt out of my depth about how to play things. Should I go along with the whole 'mum will get better' line? I'd already asked Bridget about that and her response had been unequivocal: no point in stressing Abby about the future till we knew just how bad things were likely to be. But wouldn't some preparation help? Wouldn't opening her mind to a number of possible scenarios be a useful way of drip-feeding the reality into her head? Given how her anxiety was affecting her – the obsessive cleaning, the terror of germs, the increasing social isolation – might it not be better to address the reality sooner rather than later? Perhaps I needed to call John and talk it over with him in the morning – after all, he might not even be up to speed with the medical developments.

And that 'perhaps' was soon to be upgraded to a 'definitely'. After a quiet tea during which Abby spent most of her time pushing her uneaten food around her plate and tapping her knife against her plate rim, I suggested she head up to bed, snuggle down and watch one of her new DVDs, which she seemed keener on doing than sharing the sofa with me. It was a treat to watch TV in bed in our house – particularly on a school night because, for the kids I usually had on the programme anyway, time watching DVDs or TV was a privilege they had to earn as part of the rewards system. It was a key component of the behaviour modification approach.

But an hour in I was still concerned about how poor Abby was feeling. However good it had been to clear the air with her mum, I knew she'd probably still be unsettled and upset. That was the problem when children were expected to be carers – the terrible guilt they felt for having perfectly reasonable feelings of resentment about having to take on such an onerous responsibility at such a young age. Her little rant at her mum would surely still be playing on her mind.

Armed with a glass of milk in one hand and a sandwich in the other, I couldn't knock on the bedroom door when I got up there. Instead I called out a 'hi', and pushed it open with my backside. The room was in flickering darkness, the bedside lamp off – Abby would no more leave an unnecessary light on than fly – and the only light was coming from the television. And though the film was a musical and the volume quite high, I wondered, from the mound under the covers, if she was already asleep.

I crossed the room to put the drink and sandwich down on the bedside table, but had to make space for it: there were half a dozen other DVDs stacked up there, and – to my great surprise – my kitchen scissors. For an instant I froze – how had she got them? Why had she taken them? What had she done to herself? I had seen enough damaged children for it to set alarm bells ringing in my head. I quickly put down the glass and plate and turned my attention to the bed.

'Abby, love?' I began, starting to lift the covers that concealed her, but just as I did so, the game obviously up, she stopped feigning sleep and pushed them off herself. She was busy trying to yank down the sleeves of her dressing gown, and I looked anxiously for any grisly signs of injury.

I could only see wetness on her face, however, and reached across to switch on the bedside lamp. 'Sweetie,' I said gently, sitting down on the bed, 'what are you doing?'

Abby swallowed before answering, her throat clearly catching. Judging by the look of her eyes, which were red and puffy, she'd been crying hard for some time. I reached for the milk. 'Here sweetie. Have a drink of this,' I said. And it was in passing it to her that I noticed some bits of fabric in the bed with her.

I reached for one. It looked familiar. Like part of a sock. 'What's this, love?' I asked her. Fresh tears welled in her eyes.

'I was just making bandages,' she whispered, gulping back further sobs. Once again, I heard alarm bells.

'Bandages?' I asked, confused 'Why? Are you hurt?'
She shook her head.

'Where?' I said. 'Where did you need the bandages?' I remembered the way she'd hastily pulled her sleeves down. 'On your arms? Is that it? Can I see?'

Abby was a good girl, who came from what was clearly a disciplined, loving home, however dysfunctional it might be. There was no part of her that would let her deny such a request from an adult. She duly rolled back one of her sleeves, the tears plopping onto the back of her hand as she did so.

'Shhh, it's all right, sweetheart. Don't cry ...'

'I *have* to wear them.' She gulped the words out. 'To keep my bones safe.'

'Your bones safe?'

'Or they might go like Mummy's.'

She'd now pulled the sleeve up sufficiently for me to see that – to my relief – she'd not harmed herself at all. Quite the contrary. She'd cut the toes out of some school socks to wear as 'arm bandages'. She had also cut the feet out of some woolly tights, she explained, which she was wearing under her pyjama bottoms, to 'protect' her leg bones from breaking.

'I'm sorry I took your scissors,' she said, sobbing. 'I wasn't going to steal them. I would have put them back, I promise. It's just that I couldn't bear it …' She took the milk I again proffered and drank thirstily. 'My proper ones are at home, you see, and I can't bear it. I can't sleep without my bandages. It makes me so scared. And I just lie in bed awake all night long, thinking about everything. And now Mummy's so wobbly … and I just *knew* it would happen. And now it *has* happened. It's happened to her, just like I knew it would. And now she's smashed all her bones and she can't even *walk* …'

'Oh, love,' I soothed, putting my arms round her and trying to still her once-again heaving shoulders. 'Don't worry about the scissors. But I wish you'd told me. We could have had them fetched for you, couldn't we? We still can. Promise me you'll tell me if there's anything else you need, won't you? But you know, what happened to Mummy, that was just one of those things. She fell awkwardly, that's all. And you're young and you're strong, and you really don't need to worry about your bones. Your bones are fine. They won't go wobbly.' I looked at the empty glass. 'Not with all this milk you're drinking, eh?'

I hugged her tighter, feeling absurdly relieved not to be dealing with what experience had shown me time and again I might well have been. I didn't know how the notion had lodged itself in her psyche – something else she'd read? But no wonder, with her mother's injury, that it was frightening her now, bless her. Nonetheless I was still relieved, because in the grand scheme of things her 'bandages' were harmless, just a form of comfort item really, such as a teddy was, or the corner of a blanket or a favourite doll. If she slept better wearing them, particularly at a stressful time, who was I to stop her? 'But if you want to wear them,' I reassured her, 'that's just fine by me, okay?'

Once I'd settled her, I took the scissors back down, feeling at least reassured that it was out in the open. It had obviously been really bothering her since she'd heard about her mum's fracture. And apart from anything else, she must have been chronically sleep deprived for years. No wonder she'd developed so many funny little ways. Classic anxiety symptoms, basically. I felt better, thinking it through. Perhaps, now she'd got new 'bandages', she'd find things easier to deal with.

But, of course, that would have been way too simple.

Chapter 10

Being a foster carer requires lots of skills, obviously, parenting skills chief among them. And it was certainly true that my years dealing with troubled kids in the local comprehensive had given me some solid experience on which to build. And we hadn't come into fostering blind, either. Mike and I had undergone several months of specialist training to equip us to deal with some pretty challenging children on our behaviour-modification programme.

And, as Sarah's occupational therapist, Chelsea, had pointed out, I'd already seen – and helped – my fair share of children with difficult behaviours. But I was about to discover a big gap in my knowledge, where children like Abby were concerned. It seemed I'd been going about everything all wrong.

Along with the first flush of jauntily nodding daffodils in my pretty new garden, Monday morning saw me make a mental note to get in touch with John about Sarah's condition, but before I'd had a chance to sit down and call him, it was worrying news about Abby that was first to reach my ears.

'I don't want to worry you,' said Mr Elliot on the phone (which was why I knew I should), 'but we're becoming a little concerned about Abby.'

I looked at the kitchen clock – it must have been just after playtime, and I wondered what his concerns could be; she'd barely been there an hour. And she'd trotted off happily enough, as far as I could see, having presumably slept a little better in her 'bandages'.

'Oh, dear,' I said. 'What's happened?'

'Nothing major,' he reassured me. 'You don't need to come and fetch her, or anything like that. She's fine. It's just that we've noticed lately that she's spending more time in the toilets than in the classroom – I'd made a note to give you a call this week in any case. She's been popping to the loo, oh, half a dozen times or so per lesson. And it's getting worse. I was chatting to one of my colleagues earlier, and it seems it's not just lesson time, either – she seems to spend much of the break times in the girls' toilets too. So of course our first thought was that perhaps she had some sort of stomach upset, or something. Or just – well, you know what girls this age can be like, I'm sure, what with approaching puberty and so on. And, of course, she's always been solitary, as we've already discussed. But this seems to be all about washing her hands more than anything. It seems she's developed some sort of real phobia about getting dirty – she confessed to my colleague that she worries about touching the backs of chairs, sharing crayons with the other children and so on, and it definitely seems to be getting worse. Have you noticed anything similar at home?'

I told him I had, and recounted the tetanus anxiety. 'And she's certainly a clean freak,' I added, 'as I think I mentioned when we spoke before. Not really surprising, given what we know of the situation at home.'

'I did wonder about that,' Mr Elliot said. 'And, given all the upset, whether this might all be anxiety related.'

About which I definitely agreed. 'I'm sure it is,' I said. 'She's also become very anxious about touching doorknobs and so on.'

'Yes, we noticed that too. And, of course, this morning ...'

'What actually happened?'

'Oh, forgive me,' he said. 'Like I said, it's nothing terrible. But we *are* concerned about it escalating further. The children were working with modroc this morning – it's a kind of modelling material impregnated with plaster of Paris. You might have come across it – and she became so distressed about touching it – even going *near* it – that I had to take her out of the class in the end, just to calm her down.'

'That fits,' I said. 'She really can't bear to be dirty. But, as you say, there's dirty and there's dirty ...'

'Well, exactly. And once it starts interfering with normal school activities, of course ... Anyway, I've just had a chat with the head, and we're both of a mind. What with all the hand washing and her fastidiousness generally, we were wondering if it might be developing into some kind of obsession for her, and we thought we ought to let you know our concerns. Perhaps you'd like to pop in and discuss it with us at some point? And that it might be something you'd want to mention to her GP?'

I knew that, in part, the school were probably keen to redress the balance after having been so, well, hoodwinked, for want of a better word, about just how bad things were at home for Abby, but even so I could tell Mr Elliot was genuinely concerned. And everything he'd said *had* struck a chord with me. Abby washed her hands endlessly. She was so stressed about being dirty ... It was then that I had a small 'eureka' moment. Handwashing. Obsessions about *handwashing* ... Of course! Wasn't that *the* classic symptom in people with obsessive-compulsive disorder? That and – I dredged my brain for facts – worrying that the gas had been left on? I could have kicked myself. Why on earth hadn't I connected the two? And the lights, it now occurred to me – Abby was definitely obsessive about lights. And now I was beginning to see it all differently. Was *that* what was happening? Was it more than just her anxiety about hygiene and cleanliness? Had it gone beyond that now – was Abby developing OCD?

I didn't discuss all this with Mr Elliot right there and then. I just told him I'd take some advice from social services and get back to him. Which I did need to do. If things were as bad as Mr Elliot was suggesting, I certainly needed to do *something*. I was due to be calling John Fulshaw anyway, and could perhaps call Dr Shackleton as well, though as Abby was presumably still registered with her own GP it might be better to go via Bridget – she'd presumably know who Abby's own doctor was. I rang off and called John, but he was out of the office, so, in the meantime, I did what I usually do in such circumstances: I opened my laptop, updated my log and did a bit of Googling.

Of course, as soon as I began looking at OCD websites, it seemed clearer than ever that Abby was showing signs of developing the condition as a result of her current stress. In theory, at least. I actually had no way of knowing whether this was a new thing or not. Given her home circumstances, it might have been a part of her make-up for a long time, just something that hadn't been picked up on. The business with worrying about her bones going wobbly, for instance – that had clearly been a worry for her for some time. But, thinking back over the four weeks we'd had her with us now, the kind of symptoms Mr Elliot had mentioned *were* increasing. Again, understandable, given the uncertainty around Sarah's illness. Abby had come to us expecting to be home before she knew it – but she wasn't stupid; she could see perfectly well for herself that her mother wasn't getting any better.

When the phone rang, I was glad. I knew what I was like. I'd be trawling websites for hours if left to my own devices, and I had enough wisdom to know that, in almost all cases, a little knowledge, in the hands of an amateur, was often worse than none at all. Far better to get some sensible professional input than go off half cocked. I was also anxious to speak to John about this whole Sarah situation. If Abby was going to come home from school already in a tizzy, then I wanted a clear line on how I should speak to her about her mother. Answer her questions? Spell it out? Or just continue to reassure her? It was a difficult one to call, especially as I was in the dark myself.

But it wasn't John on the phone, it was Riley.

'Jackson's party, Mum,' she began, without preamble. 'We're going to have to postpone it.'

To my shame I'd not given my grandson's party so much as half a second's thought so far this morning, despite us having already made plans to have it the following weekend.

'Why, love?' I asked, pretending I had, obviously.

'Precautionary measure,' she said briskly. 'No choice. One of Levi's pals at nursery has gone down with MRSA.'

'MRSA?' It was obviously going to be a morning of medical acronyms. And this was no nicer than the last two. 'Oh dear.'

'Quite. Oh dear is right.'

'But isn't that the one you get when you're in hospital? I didn't think you tended to get it otherwise. Nasty bug to get. Are they sure?'

'Apparently. I think the mum was in for something and has been ill with it, or something. But you know what these things are like – the usual sharp intake of breath, the mass terror of contagion, the usual "step away from that plague child!" response. Can you imagine what the average nursery school would have been like during the plague?'

'Er, empty? Aww, poor little thing. Are they very sick?'

'Bearing up, as far as I can tell. Possibly even on the mend now. But there's been another one picked up today with sickness and diarrhoea symptoms, so everyone's panicking that it's going to spread, of course. It's an emotive word, MRSA, isn't it? A bit like "nits". Everyone's stressing their little one might have caught it as well now – and yes, Mum, Levi is absolutely *fine*, before you ask, and it's not a child he's particularly close to or anything. But I just thought it made more sense to postpone Jackson's party than to have everyone cry off at the last minute – or, more pertinently, think I'm being a *deeply* irresponsible mum.'

Riley was right, of course. It was the sensible thing to do. The days when mums liked to hold chickenpox and measles parties so all the kids could get it over with were long gone. And Jackson wouldn't give a hoot. He'd only be one. This wasn't a party he'd even remember.

'It might be better in any case,' I agreed. 'Give the chance for the weather to warm up a bit. And, actually, putting it back a couple of weeks means we could hold it on Abby's birthday itself, come to think of it. If you don't mind us doing it on the Friday, that is.' And with Abby's current problems, I also thought, but didn't say, it might just be one less thing for her to get stressed about right now. 'But now I'd better get off the phone anyway. I'm waiting on a call from John Fulshaw.'

'Okay,' Riley said. 'But listen – just be sure to disinfect the phone now we've spoken to me. You know what these virulent new superbugs are like …'

'God,' I groaned, thinking how ironic her joke was under the current circumstances. 'Don't you start!'

'I know hardly anything about Sarah's current medical condition, to be honest,' John admitted, once he'd called back half an hour later and I'd given him a run-down on what Chelsea had told me about the clinical trial and the possible plans for Sarah to remain in hospital long term.

'Do you think Bridget does?' I asked him. 'I'm very conscious that Chelsea thought *I* knew. It sounds serious, doesn't it? And if she's got to go into some residential rehabilitation programme as well ... Well, it will obviously change things, won't it? Have you had any sort of update on the situation with finding relatives? What about those second cousins she mentioned? Any news there?' As I spoke it occurred to me that I'd had almost nothing in the way of updates either. Which was unusual in itself. Why not? Usually, there were more meetings than you knew what to do with. But then, Abby wasn't usual, in that she wasn't in my usual category. The kids we had mostly required loads of meetings, to plan strategies for coping with the extreme things they did, and in some cases, just to keep them from absconding, not to mention falling foul of the law.

'I'm also conscious,' I went on, 'that if that *is* what's going to happen, then Abby needs to be prepared for things properly.'

I explained about the school's worries and how I wanted to know what action John thought I should take. 'And I was wondering if I should go and see the school, or whether it's Bridget who should be speaking to them. In conjunction with Sarah, even. Though, as of this moment, we don't know what "it" even is, do we? Not definitively. I mean, normally, I'd just get on with it, and call Dr Shackleton, but do you think Bridget would want to take Abby to her own GP?'

'I'd better speak to her,' John said. 'I see no reason why you couldn't give him a call and get some general advice, I suppose, but before you make an appointment with the school or start thinking about strategies, let's see what Bridget has to say, yes? You're right. This *is* an unusual situation, in that no one here is trying to exclude Sarah from proceedings, are they? And we also know how it is with all these various protocols. Don't want you to be seen as stepping on any social service toes, eh?'

We both laughed, of course – stepped-on toes were a constant worry in my line of work – but little did I know that John's words would be coming back to haunt me, and would wipe the smile right off my face.

It's reassuringly straightforward, I think, the way the human mind works. While you're oblivious to something, you obviously don't look for it, but once something's pointed out to you, suddenly it's so *there* – you can't seem to miss it if you try.

Like being a schoolgirl, in a playground, perhaps, and your friend points out a boy she tells you fancies you. One minute you're barely aware of his existence, the next, he seems to be everywhere you go. I remembered that sort of thing happening to me more than once when I was younger. Once you know something, you can't un-know it, and it sticks in your mind.

By the time Abby returned from school, I had trawled, if not the entire internet, at least my memories of the time she'd been with us, and found Mr Elliot's concerns to be well founded. Things I'd previously attributed to force of habit, due to her circumstances (the making of endless lists, the hygiene issues, the need to turn lights off, the terror of illness), I could now see might equally be part of a pattern of an increasingly over-the-top anxiety response.

I had decided to say nothing to Abby about the incident in school that morning – that should maybe wait until I knew who was going to do what. For the same reason I'd also held off on calling Dr Shackleton. I would do as John suggested and wait for Bridget to guide me – but I *had* taken the school's worries on board, and had resolved to keep a closer eye on Abby. And, of course, as soon as I did that it all became clear. The poor child was really struggling with day-to-day living to such an extent that I couldn't believe I'd missed it.

I followed her around like a proverbial hawk over the next couple of days, and my eyes were truly opened to the extent of it. Not just one or two – *every* doorknob was opened with a sleeve, be it the front door or an interior door or the handle on a cupboard. The visits to the toilet – which I'd previously never really worried about that much (it was the other way round with most kids: will you *please* wash your hands!) happened not just here and there, to answer a call of nature, but at intervals that at first seemed inexplicably short, until you realised they immediately followed Abby doing *anything* that might be dirty, such as taking something from me – a tea towel, an apple or a pile of magazines. She'd do whatever I asked of her and then immediately disappear, and then return from the downstairs loo or, if more appropriate, the kitchen sink, having carefully washed and dried her hands. I also noticed that she didn't use my fabric towels either. In the kitchen she would wash her hands, dry them on kitchen paper, then pop the kitchen towel in the kitchen bin, using the foot pedal. The same applied in the downstairs loo – I even stood outside and listened. I would hear the flush, then the sink taps, then the rattle of the toilet roll holder for a second time and, finally, a second flush, and only then would she re-emerge.

Other things were more subtle. I recalled her hair-pulling that first evening, and began taking note of any time when she started to do it, and, to my astonishment, found that she was doing it quite consciously, and that there was a definite pattern there, too. She would pull half a dozen hairs out, line them up on the chair arm beside her, then, when she'd done that, gather the strands together and roll them into a ball.

I also noticed that the switching off of lights was equally ritualistic. It wasn't just a case of going around plunging the house into darkness. She would also switch on any light that was off, as if to check it. She'd flick it on for half a second, before switching it back off again, as if reassuring herself it really wasn't lit. She would then pat the switch plate several times, for good measure.

In short, she was in a state and it was a state that was definitely worsening. And I wanted some guidance on how to help her. So when I got an email from Bridget, finally, on the Wednesday, I felt frustrated. The email was brief. And ironic. *Dear Casey*, it read, *apologies for being so slow to come back to you. I've been off with some dreadful bug – ugh! – but am now back on the case. Are you free for me to pop in for a bit of an update next Thursday?*

'Harrumph!' I said to Mike, after I'd read it out to him. 'She hasn't even mentioned who she thinks should be updating who! And look –' I pointed. 'Next Thursday? That's more than a week away!'

Mike squeezed my shoulder. He knew what I was like. Once I'd decided on something I was like a dog with a bone. I wanted action. Not meetings next bloody Thursday.

'Ah, but perhaps she's had MRSA as well,' he quipped.

Once again, I laughed. But inside I was still harrumphing. Stuff it, I *would* call Dr Shackleton.

Chapter 11

Dr Shackleton, our local GP, has always been a godsend. He's been the family doctor since before Riley was born, and even though our recent house move meant we were a little bit outside his area there was no way I'd consider leaving his surgery unless physically restrained from going there.

Kids in foster care sometimes retain their own GP, and others not – it depends on the individual circumstances. This was certainly true of the children we'd had so far. Where a child was to be with us long term, it obviously made sense to get their notes transferred to him – which he was graciously accepting of – and in others, where it was short term or there was some other compelling reason, the child would continue with the practice they already had.

Dr Shackleton was also wonderful because he was such a great supporter of what Mike and I did. He'd been particularly invaluable in helping us with one of our earlier foster children, Sophia, who had a rare hormonal disorder called Addison's disease. It had been a lifeline more than once to have him at the end of the phone.

Though I obviously couldn't speak to him specifically about Abby's case, I could at least get an overview of what her symptoms might mean and, most importantly, how to help her manage them. I was particularly concerned about how it was affecting her at school. She had enough to deal with without becoming even more ostracised than she already was. I called the surgery the morning after receiving Bridget's email and was able to book a quick telephone consultation for the end of morning surgery, so I could at least talk the problems I'd seen through with him.

And he was predictably helpful.

'I think you're spot on,' he agreed. 'This sounds very much like stress-related OCD. And the good news is that very often it's only temporary, particularly when it manifests in children. It can run in families, and it tends to afflict the already anxious – it's often a trigger such as you've described that tips the person over into a place where they can no longer manage those anxieties, after which it's particularly good at feeding off itself – it's the enemy within, so to speak. And from what you describe that's what seems to be happening here. Though, on a more positive note, you may well find it begins to settle down once she gets more used to her new living arrangements.'

Which were completely up in the air, truth be told. Who knew what was going to happen to her? No one, right now, it seemed. But once we did – well, that was at least encouraging. 'That's reassuring to hear,' I said. 'Because right now it seems to be going the other way. She's been with us over a month now, and though I reasoned it might be partly because it's only now I've really started noticing, the compulsions seem to be getting worse daily.' And that was, literally, what seemed to be happening. I'd now caught her several times tapping her fingers on all the door frames – as if she couldn't walk through one before doing so. 'I keep reassuring her,' I told him. 'I don't try to stop her doing what she needs to do – far from it. If she needs to polish the doorknobs, or tap things, or wear her special "bandages", then I've let her …'

'Ah,' said Dr Shackleton, 'that's exactly what you shouldn't do.'

Now I was confused. Wouldn't stopping her make her even more anxious? 'But I thought drawing attention to a behaviour was the last thing I should be doing,' I said. 'Isn't that tantamount to reinforcing it?'

'In many cases, yes, obviously. But there's a subtle difference here. With errant toddlers and attention-seeking teenagers, of course that's true. In cases like that, you're absolutely right. You *are* reinforcing a behaviour, which, in the case of an undesirable, attention-seeking behaviour – such as a tantrum or a rant – is obviously the last thing you want to do. Reinforce the good, don't reward the bad with attention, and so on. But this is different. With compulsions – which are essentially rituals employed to minimise feelings of acute fear or anxiety, as opposed to being used to get the child's own way – the trick is to *confront* them. You'll have heard the expression 'feel the fear and do it anyway', no doubt?'

'One of my mottos, as it happens.'

'Well, that's what it's all about. And it's the opposite of what an anxious OCD sufferer does. They feel the fear and "run away" from what frightens them. And the "running away" of course – which is what they're doing when they adopt all these little tics – just makes the fear feel bigger next time. So it might start with tapping something once, and then escalate to several times, or be augmented by additional rituals, till in the end it becomes so elaborate and frequent that it's almost impossible to function. You see what I'm saying?'

'Yes, I get that.'

'Well, OCD is an extreme form of that. What happens to the OCD sufferer is that, under stress that perhaps rational fear gets blown up into something so big as to be difficult to manage. So, in this case, say Abby has this fear of getting sick. Perfectly understandable given what you describe of her childhood environment, but now she has to deal with the additional stress of having to leave her mother and go and live with strangers – losing all her reassuring routines and rituals behind in the process – so now she feels the fear and finds it unbearable. Hence the obsessions and compulsions. In simple terms, she can't avoid her current circumstances, so she has found ways to reduce her anxiety about them, by endless hand washing, germ obliteration and so on.

'Of course, there's a lot more to it than that,' he went on. 'The other main thing that happens is that the brain finds all sorts of clever ways to alleviate anxiety – and that's where repetitive tics come in – the light switch flicking and hair pulling you mentioned. Patients often can't explain why they do some of these things, except to report that it makes them feel better. Again, it's just a way of controlling their fears. If I turn round on the spot three times – to pick something at random – the horrible feelings of dread in my head go away.'

This was beginning to make sense to me now. 'Ah, I get it. So I shouldn't be indulging them, then. I should be trying to stop them. Intervening.'

'Exactly. To accept tics as being "normal" is reinforcing them, obviously. It's like saying "Go ahead – you're right to be afraid of the thing that scares you" because that's what it's about. An irrational obsession. So, generally speaking, you need to be doing the opposite. Not in a traumatising way, obviously – just gently encouraging her to confront her fears and so shrink them down to a rational size. It's a bit like managing phobias. First she needs to be exposed to the things that frighten her, so she breaks that cycle of fear and avoidance. Second, she needs to be distracted from ritual tics – gently steered away from doing them. In both cases it's all about her re-learning the associations she's made – having it reinforced instead that if she touches a door handle or a chair back she's not going to die, and that if she doesn't perform her tics then nothing bad is going to happen to either her or her loved ones – in this case, her mother. Again, I'm grossly over-simplifying, but that's the gist of it. That help?'

'Immeasurably,' I said. 'Wow, I'm certainly learning in this job, eh?'

'Life is short, the art long, as we medics are wont to say. Another useful mantra for you, Casey!'

I felt much better having spoken to Dr Shackleton. And now I was armed with more information about the logic of the disorder – and, in its own perverse way, it *was* logical – I felt better equipped to help Abby start to manage it. Once I'd spoken to Bridget, of course (and we had a clearer sense of what might happen in the longer term), maybe some professional intervention might be appropriate, in the form of a course of cognitive behavioural therapy, to help her deal with it. Or maybe all would be well, and she and Sarah would go home and, magically, the symptoms would disappear. But I wasn't holding my breath, and right now she needed support, so in the meantime I could practise my own small interventions – or ERP routine, as Dr Shackleton had called it: exposure and ritual prevention.

For poor Abby, though, this must have felt like another great weight on her shoulders, which were already buckling under the strain.

'You know what?' I said to her, the afternoon after I'd spoken to Dr Shackleton. 'I'm starving. And Mike's working late, so tea's going to be *ages* away yet. So how about we go and choose a cake from the cake counter?'

We were in the supermarket, straight after school, which had already thrown her somewhat. Her ritual – as I now realised it to be – hadn't varied since she'd come to us. She would come in, go into the downstairs loo, wash her hands, straight upstairs, change out of her uniform, then wash her hands again upstairs, then come down again, at which point I'd make her a snack. The only times that hadn't happened were when we'd gone to the hospital, when I'd taken something for her to eat on the way there. And, of course, now I realised that on neither occasion had she eaten it. I'd naturally put it down to the emotion of seeing her mum, but now I realised it was actually more complicated than that.

She shook her head now. 'I'm not hungry. I mean, you get one if you want to.'

'But surely you must be,' I urged, heading towards the bakery anyway. 'You've had nothing since lunchtime.' And she'd probably eaten very little of that, either, it occurred to me. And I doubted she'd be monitored that closely over lunch – the older juniors generally didn't tend to be.

'Really,' she persisted. 'I'm fine, Casey, honest. But you get one if you want one.'

I pulled a sad face. 'Oh, *please*,' I said. We'd reached the counter by now. 'I'll feel like *such* a greedy pig if you don't have one as well. Just a little fairy cake or something? Or a cookie? They look nice. Or an iced bun perhaps?'

I was being horribly manipulative, and I knew it. Poor Abby would be torn now between doing as I had asked and the stress of the situation, and I knew how much of a tussle must be going on in her head. Other kids would just refuse point blank to do something they didn't want to, but I knew for Abby, who wasn't used to being disobedient or contrary, this would be a real poser. I just hoped her urge to do what was asked of her would win out.

I leaned towards the trolley, which I'd made her push for me, citing a blister I'd got scrubbing the garden furniture. Like a school chair, or a public door handle, it might have been previously pushed by anyone, and having to touch it was already upsetting her equilibrium. 'Sweetheart,' I said gently. 'Go on. Please. For me? I worry about you, you know. I'm sure you're not eating enough. And I'll feel awful if we go to visit Mummy on Friday and she starts worrying that you've been losing weight. *Awful.*'

This spot of emotional blackmail seemed to clinch it. She mumbled an okay and shyly pointed to the pile of hot cross buns, and within ten minutes we'd gone through the checkout with our bits of shopping, and I suggested we munch our cakes once we'd returned to the car. That way, I'd calculated, there would be no chance for her to fly off and do what she desperately wanted to – wash her hands. And as I'd told her not to bring her backpack – telling her we'd be there and back in no time – she didn't even have recourse to the little bottle of anti-bacterial gel I'd recently discovered she kept in there.

'How nice was *that*?' I enthused, once I'd chomped my way through an uncharacteristically-decadent-for-four p.m. éclair. Abby had finished her bun as well – as I'd suspected, she'd been ravenous – but now wore an expression of great anxiety about what to do next. I switched the engine on, to forestall any requests to pop back and use the toilets, and as I reversed out of the parking space and swung the car round to leave the car park I marvelled on what a complex and powerful thing the human psyche was. How much of her day was governed, I wondered, by trying to organise every tiny detail so she could minimise such awful stress? It must have been so debilitating. No wonder she found school so challenging. Ditto living with us and losing so much of that control. One major factor in her previous living arrangements, I realised, would have been that she could give in to these compulsions and organise her life to do so. Her mother – probably preoccupied with her own debilitating illness – had quite possibly not even noticed.

I glanced across at Abby. She was sitting with one hand in her lap now, the other once again plucking single strands of hair from her scalp. 'You know, sweetheart,' I said, deciding this might be a good place to broach it, 'nothing bad is going to happen because you haven't washed your hands.'

The effect was instant. Her hand flew away from her temple and the hairs she'd pulled out so far were brushed from her lap. 'I don't ...' she began. 'I mean ... um ... erm ... what do you mean, Casey?'

'I mean,' I said, joining the crawling early rush-hour traffic – there was a reason I didn't generally do a supermarket run after school – 'that I understand how you worry about things, sweetie. Germs and so on. Getting sick. I absolutely understand why you might be worried about that. And yes, you're right – the world is just full of germs, isn't it? Just like it's full of people. But, trust me, the chances of catching a bad one – one that'll make you poorly – are really tiny, you know. *Tiny*. Tinier even than winning the lottery. I mean, it's obviously sensible to wash your hands before your tea – that's just good hygiene. But sometimes you have to relax and trust that nothing bad will happen. I've eaten that many cakes, from that many different baker-ies down the years, and look at me!' I patted my stomach. 'The only harm that's come to me has been the harm to my waistline …' Which, to my relief, at least raised a suspicion of a smile. 'So that's what you have to do,' I said. 'You have to tell yourself that *nothing bad will happen*. And keep saying it to yourself till the other bit of you *believes* it. Maybe try that for me, hmm?'

Abby didn't look convinced, even though she did nod her acknowledgement, and once we were home she bolted straight for the loo, as I'd expected. This time I didn't try to stop her. But neither did I let up on my subtle pressure to challenge her obsessions. On the contrary. Over the next couple of days I gently stepped it up. Not overtly – it seemed too much too soon to start actually interrogating her about things like flicking the light switches and patting the door frames – but in the sense that I tried to make it just that little more difficult for her to give in to them. I began making it harder for her to avoid touching door handles, for instance, having noticed, as with the hair, that it mattered to her that we *didn't* notice when she did things like covering her hand with her sleeve to open them. If we were around, and she had no choice, she would always try to compensate – by immediately going off 'to the loo' to wash her hands. So I'd have her open a door for me, saying my hands were full or something, and then herd her off into another room on some pretext or other, so that she would have to wait for another hand-washing opportunity. I would similarly tend to hover around light switches, and forestall her in flicking them on and off. One thing, I thought wryly, would be a big dip in the electricity bills. The Watson house had never been such a bastion of green living.

It wasn't plain sailing – I could see that it was actually adding to her anxiety, but though it upset me to see that, I trusted Dr Shackleton. Over time, I hoped it would help. I was also anxious to be proactive rather than just reactive. My role as a foster carer was to provide an environment that helped the kids in my care to feel better, not worse, and what the school had said – that since we'd last spoken she seemed to have got quite a *lot* worse – went against everything Mike and I set out to do. I knew it wasn't strictly our fault – Abby had come from somewhere she was cherished, not neglected, where normally the opposite was true – but, even so, it definitely concentrated my mind. I could accept the fact that Abby wanted nothing more than to be home again, and that was what we all wanted too, however unlikely that was currently looking. But in the meantime, the very last thing *I* wanted was to take her to see Sarah and give Sarah any reason to worry about *her*.

Which was a reasonable enough aim, I thought. Wasn't it?

Chapter 12

In the end, we didn't go and visit Sarah on the Friday. I took a call from Bridget late that morning. The hospital had called her to tell her that Sarah was exhausted, having had daily physio for the past few days, and that she'd also been having a series of drug infusions, which had been really knocking her for six. As a consequence they'd all agreed that perhaps it would be counter-productive for Abby to go and visit her while she was so far from her best.

'Given how distressing it was for them both last time,' Bridget finished. 'Sarah will call Abby tonight at some point, obviously. But we wondered if you could take her in on Sunday instead. Give Sarah a day to recover. If that's not going to inconvenience you too much?'

'Not at all,' I reassured her, thinking how, actually, it was just as well Jackson's party had been cancelled, as fitting in both would have been something of a struggle. At the same time, my heart was plummeting towards my boots. Poor

Abby. The one thing I knew was keeping her going was the knowledge that she would be seeing her mum again this afternoon. Instead, I'd have to break bad news when she arrived home from school.

And she was every bit as upset as I'd expected her to be. I'd seen her arrival from the kitchen window, and she'd fairly skipped up the path – looking the brightest she'd done in days. I hated having to burst her fragile bubble.

'Why does she keep *doing* this!' she railed at me now, her eyes filling with tears immediately, as I explained that we wouldn't now be going to the hospital to visit Mummy after all. 'She told me she was feeling better. She *told* me! She *promised*!'

I pulled Abby towards me, but she struggled to get out of my grasp, and thundered up the stairs to her bedroom. I heard the door slam behind her and, as I followed her up, I also heard various thumps and bangs starting up. She was clearly venting her distress at the furniture. Which might be no bad thing, I decided, as I reached the landing. I wasn't fazed – as far as explosions of temper went, Abby's was relatively minor compared to some I'd had to deal with, and dealing with distressed children was all part of the job in our line of work. But for Abby it was quite a big deal to lose control like this; it wasn't something I'd so far seen from her and I'd bet my last farthing that having childish tantrums, for any of the usual childish reasons, would have been something she'd stopped doing very early on. She'd had to grow up much too fast, in order to care for her mother.

I knocked on the door, feeling a wave of irritation at Sarah. Much as I tried to be politically correct about the situation – and I did feel pretty guilty for even thinking it – I couldn't help thinking that Abby's not being allowed to see her had been decided for all the wrong reasons. However difficult it would be for Abby to see Sarah so poorly, surely not being allowed to see her at all was far worse. After all, she'd been caring for her sick mother for years now. And in that time she would surely have seen her in a pretty bad way, wouldn't she? She used the words 'relapse' and 'remission'; she knew the illness. More than most, in fact, me included – because she'd been living with it, day in, day out. And I didn't doubt she knew how things stood. No, I thought, as I softly knocked on her door, this was a bad call. This was just shutting her out, which wasn't helping her one bit. Surely her mother – who must be aware what an anxious child she was – must have known that?

There was no response, just the sound of the continuing thumps and bumps. Was she kicking the chest of drawers? Well, if so, so what? They could take it. It was the same chest of drawers I'd bought when we first started fostering, and had already put up with plenty. It would survive. I turned the handle and opened the bedroom door to find I'd been right. Abby was laying into the chest of drawers with one foot and thumping it at the same time with one of her cushions – a *Glee* one I'd found in the supermarket recently, on special offer, being left-over Christmas stock.

'Oh, sweetheart,' I said to her. 'I'm so sorry, I really am. But it's only going to be a couple of days. And Mummy's going to phone you later, so at least you'll get to chat to her ...'

'I didn't want to see her anyway,' Abby railed at me, 'and I don't want to talk to her!' She flung the cushion back on the bed and angrily wiped the back of her hand across her tear-stained face. 'She obviously doesn't need me to look after her any more, and that's fine. That's just *fine*.' She spat the last word out. I could see spittle arc across the space between us. I'd not seen her furious like this before, but I decided it would probably be cathartic, even though it was heartbreaking to hear.

'You know that's not true,' I said gently. 'Of *course* she needs you. She *loves* you, Abby.'

'No she doesn't!'

'Sweetheart, she *does*. She loves you more than anything or anyone in the whole world. And what she most needs is to know that you're okay while you can't be with her. I'm sure you're on her mind every minute of every day.'

Abby's expression remained one of angry rejection. 'No, I'm not! If I was, she'd let me go and *see* her! She's just forgotten about me, now she doesn't need me to make her food and wash her clothes and keep the house tidy for her! She doesn't even care that it's going to be getting so filthy!'

'Sweetheart, that doesn't matter. The house can be cleaned. What matters is that Mummy gets properly looked after by the doctors and nurses. That they do the very best they can to make this horrible illness she has ...' I grasped for words – 'go away' were entirely the wrong ones. '... beat it,' I plumped for. 'Try to beat it a little better. So she's got a chance of getting home again and being more independent. So that the two of you can be together again. Get back to being a family ...'

The word seemed to inflame her anger further. 'We're *not* a family!' she yelled at me. 'How can we ever be called a family?! Everyone else has daddies and brothers and sisters and cousins and nannies and granddads and everything!' she spat. 'I don't have *anything*! I don't have anyone in the *world* now!'

She threw herself down on the bed then, her whole body overcome with huge, racking sobs. I sat down beside her, and tried to envelope her. 'You *are* a family,' I persisted, speaking quietly into her ear. 'You're your mummy's little girl, and that *makes* you a family. Yes, a small family, compared with some, but still a family. Still unbreakable. Family's not about numbers anyway. It's about love. And I know how much your mummy loves you. And how much you love her too. And you know, Abby, I've looked after lots of children, and some of them don't even *have* mummies. And some of them have mummies who don't love them anything like as much as yours does. Mummies who don't cuddle them or care about them. Mummies who don't even want to *know* them. That's not *your* mummy, is it?' I stroked her hair. It was wet around the temples, where she'd been perspiring from all the flailing around. 'Why do you think Mummy was so upset last time we visited her, hmm? Because she misses you so much, and can hardly bear that she's not with you ...' I had slid my fingers beneath her hair now, pulling it back from where it was sticking to her face, to loop around her ear. I was just about to speak again when her hand flew up and clamped mine. 'What, sweetheart?' I said, shocked. 'What's the matter? Did I scratch you with my nail?'

Abby wriggled up to a sitting position, freeing my hand and now clamping her own firmly to her temple. But why? What was she hiding? What didn't she want me to see? 'Abby,' I tried again. 'What are you doing? Why've you got your hand there?'

'Nothing,' she said, straightening up. 'I just didn't want you to ...'

'*What*? Love, if it's nothing, then why don't you want me to see it?'

She looked agitated again, shaking her head now. What was she trying to hide from me? 'Abby,' I said, 'you know, you might as well let me see it, whatever it is. I'm going to get to see it eventually, so –'

'Oh, for God's sake! OKAY!' She stepped towards me, thrusting her face at me and pouting. Then she turned sideways and yanked the hair back out of the way. 'There!' she said. '*That's* what it is. Are you happy now?'

It didn't need much looking at, now she'd scraped the hair away from it. It was a bald patch, pink and stark, just slightly behind her ear. A completely bald patch, about two inches in diameter. Shiny. Substantially bigger than a ten pence piece.

I was shocked. Oh, yes, I'd seen lots of things that had shocked me over the years, and, no, in comparison, this wasn't *that* shocking. Yet it still was. Because *why the hell hadn't I spotted it?* Why hadn't I thought about all her hair pulling and the obvious result of it? Why hadn't I realised just how bad it was?

I held her head in both hands and inspected it more closely. And it extended. The hair around it was thin and sparse as well. 'Did this fall out?' I asked her, even though I already knew it probably hadn't. She shook her head, confirming it. 'This is the place where you *pull* your hair out, isn't it?' Now she nodded. And I cursed myself again for not making the mental leap about what we'd seen her doing, not *doing* something about it, before it came to this. It was so big – and now so obvious – yet she'd still managed to keep it hidden from me. 'Has it been like this for long?' I asked.

Abby shook her head. 'Only a little,' she said in a small voice. 'But it's just got so ... so ... It's just that I can't seem to stop doing it. I don't even realise I'm doing it ... except I do ...' Her eyes glistened with fresh tears.

And then she'd carefully cover it up, I thought, every single day, by neatly pulling her hair into bunches, or plaits. Never a pony tail. Always bunches, always plaits. And I recalled that she also used those little spring clips you got in Claire's Accessories. So that even when it wasn't safely covered up by plaits or bunches, she could still hide it, by clipping her hair in place, to hold it down.

I took her hands in my own now and made her hold my gaze. 'We can get you some help for this,' I said. 'We can get someone – a special doctor, who knows about the things people sometimes do when they're anxious – someone who can help you stop doing this, okay? And then it will grow back again –'

'Will it?' she asked, her eyes wide.

'Of course it will!' I told her, trying to pack my voice with confidence and authority. Because it would do. I was sure of it. As sure as I could be, anyway. I racked my brains. This was different from stress-induced alopecia. This had another name. And it would *surely* grow back. Why wouldn't it? If it were caught in time. 'Of, *course* it will,' I said again, firmly.

Abby nodded. She looked so tired, and so forlorn. I put my arms round her. 'When I speak to Bridget next week, we'll get it all organised for you, okay? Someone you can talk to, who understands. And who can help you with all of it. Help you stop worrying about germs, and being frightened. And feeling you can't stop yourself pulling your hair out, and having to wash your hands all the time … They can do that, you know.' I tapped my own temple. 'Because they're clever. And they speak to lots of children who have your problems. And they know just what pesky things our minds are. Always going off half-cocked, on their own wild and crazy schemes of bonkersness …'

This at last elicited something of a smile from her. She probably felt better, I decided, having got some of this off her chest. Time to tuck it away again now, at least for a bit. Enough for one day. 'But right now,' I said firmly. 'I think we could both do with some R and R, eh? So how about we go downstairs, and I'll make us both some crumpets, with *lashings* of chocolate spread on them, and then the two of us will sit down and watch one of those movies together, hmm? It'll be a couple of hours till Mike's home, so we've got plenty of time. And guess what? Kieron's coming over later, because Lauren's out with her girl-friends, so maybe we can get some games out or some-thing later on, yes?'

At the mention of Kieron, I was pleased to see a flicker of interest. And once again it occurred to me how much they were on the same wavelength. For completely differ-ent reasons, of course, but there was something about Kieron's need for order and love of ritual that seemed to tap into Abby's psyche and calm her down. I'd just better make sure I was right about him coming. And if Sarah *didn't* flipping call … *No*, I thought, heading the thought off before I thought it. *Not your department. Just concentrate on Abby*.

I let her go and wash her hands then. She had had enough stress today, and I knew denying her the chance to do so would only give her a load more. God, though, I thought, how had I missed that? Crazy schemes of bonkersness was just about right. I made a mental note to do a bit more Googling.

'I bring exciting news!' Kieron announced, almost as soon as he'd arrived. 'Week tomorrow. 9 a.m. kick-off. The offi-cial Saturday cupcakeathon at *Truly Scrumptious*! A cupcake for all seasons and all reasons in every colour, to raise money for Sport Relief. I have the flyers, and I'm not afraid to use them!'

Kieron and Bob had arrived just as the credits were rolling on *High School Musical*, by which time Abby, exhausted after the afternoon's disclosures, had watched a third of the film, fallen asleep on me, and then woken up in time to watch the end. Which didn't matter. No doubt she'd watch it again at some point.

And Mike would be home soon, so we had to get cracking. We would have our favourite, I'd decided, my special family recipe for corned-beef hash. Special, on account of there needing to be no onions, but plenty of baked beans mixed in with the potatoes, which was the way Kieron liked it. And, it turned out, happily Abby did too.

The three of us trooped into the kitchen, accompanied by Bob. Abby really did look so much brighter now, and I was pleased.

'The what?' I asked. 'The Cupathon? What's a cupathon?'

'Cup*cake*athon,' Kieron corrected. 'At Auntie Donna's. Mum, you *know*.'

Kerplunk. The penny dropped. I pulled a bag of potatoes from my veg rack. Abby was already bustling around, washing her hands again and donning her little pinny. I noticed she marched around like a surgeon scrubbed up for an operation when Bob was around. Elbows up, out of licking range. 'I'll do those,' she said, as I plonked the potatoes on the worktop. She loved humdrum domestic tasks the same way other girls loved Justin Beiber, and now I was seeing things with more clinical eyes I realised that they were perhaps a coping mechanism of their own.

'Of course,' I said to Kieron. 'You know, I'd forgotten all about that. It's next weekend, then, is it? God, that seems to have come around fast.'

It had too. My own life having been so full on just recently – what with moving house after so long, saying goodbye to Spencer and getting Abby – I'd had little time, since the Christmas celebrations, for extended family. But in the meantime my younger sister, Donna, had had something of a life-change herself. Like our parents, she'd started out in the catering business, but after a gap for children, and some less full-on 9 to 5 employment over in Ireland, where my brother-in-law was from, she'd got the bug again to run her own business. Last summer she'd bought the lease on a little café close to the town centre, which she'd styled to look like a Victorian tearoom. She was an expert, of course – her previous place had thrived – and it was already doing far better than even she had imagined. It was all pretty, mismatched floral china, lace doilies and crisp tablecloths – and, as far as fashion went, right on the button.

It wasn't Kieron's natural habitat – the very opposite of it, really (Kieron didn't like mismatched anything), but while he was doing his training as a youth worker he was chronically short of cash, having just his bits of DJing to support him. So it suited them both for him to do a few hours down there every week – Donna because it was always nice to have family in family businesses, and Kieron because it meant he didn't starve.

It had been Kieron's idea to put on an event there to raise money for Sport Relief as well. With football being his passion, he always tried to support it, hence the big bakeathon – or 'cupcakeathon' – the following weekend, where they'd be having a bit of a party and a bake-off competition, and selling masses of 'designer' cupcakes, at a premium, to support the cause. He was even missing playing his beloved Saturday match for it – a sure mark of his commitment to it, bless him.

'Yes, it has,' he said, 'and I've got to publicise it – hence the flyers. I've also given a bunch to Riley, but perhaps you could hand a few out as well for me?'

'Sure I can,' I said. 'Perhaps you could even take some to school, Abby.'

Abby nodded. She'd got some colour back in her cheeks now and looked altogether happier.

'And we're going to be grateful,' added Kieron, 'for all offers of cupcake making, obviously. We're going to need a LOT. And I'm a rubbish baker. So I told Auntie Donna that you'd help out – seeing as it's for charity …'

'Oh, you did, did you?' I laughed.

'I know how to make cupcakes,' chimed in Abby. 'I can make some.'

'Excellent!' said Kieron, beaming. 'You are officially recruited, then. And you're going to come, right? And bring Dad and that, and Riley …'

'I'm sure Dad'll come – though probably not before eleven, obviously, as he'll be working.' Though not a minute later, mind – Saturdays had been sacrosanct ever since Kieron had joined the local kids' football league, aged twelve. In almost ten years Mike had hardly missed a match himself. 'But we'll definitely come down early and help you set things up, won't we, Abby? And – Oh hell! Hang on ...' An alarm bell had started ringing. 'What's the date this Saturday?' I glanced at the pile of flyers and groaned. 'Damn it!'

'What?' said Kieron.

I went across to the wall calendar and confirmed it. I had a training session the following Saturday. Out of town. 8 a.m. sharp. These were something I only had to do a few times a year, so it tended to slip my mind. But the bell had rung for a reason. I knew there was something about that date. The next one was taking place the following weekend. 'Attachment Theory', the calendar said. And there was no way I could un-attach myself from it. 'I've got my foster training this Saturday morning,' I explained. 'Typical! I mean I'll be done by 3, so I could get there eventually, and show my face, but ... actually, there's a thought.' I glanced at Abby. Saturday. No school. I'd need to find some respite care for her, too, at least till Mike got home.

That would be the usual way you'd do it, anyway, if you needed a babysitter for a foster child, but this was short notice, and for such a short period, it seemed hardly sensible. Plus I'd hate to have to drop her with a stranger. She was fragile enough right now. No, perhaps I'd ask Riley. I'd had both her and Kieron police-checked when we started fostering, and had them reassessed as family carers regularly. It made perfect sense, as it meant they could babysit if it was ever needed. And for them, too; since they both wanted to work in the sector eventually, it was one less thing to worry about later.

'We'll have to ask Riley if I can drop you off at hers, love,' I explained to Abby. 'You'd like that, wouldn't you? Spend some time with the little ones? And you could obviously still pop along to the cupcakeathon with them …'

'Hey, not so fast, pardner!' Kieron interrupted. 'If Abby's free, why doesn't she just come down and help *me*?'

He gave Abby a thumbs up and a wink. 'Love,' I started. 'I think it would be better …'

'No, I'd like that,' said Abby shyly. 'I could be your assistant, couldn't I?'

'And, hey,' he said, pointing. 'You even have your own pinny. And I know for a fact that you are an ace washer-upper. Do you take payment in cupcakes?' Abby grinned. 'Mum,' he said, turning back to me now, 'you know it makes sense.'

I thought for all of two seconds. Of *course* it made sense. She'd love it down there. And I knew Donna wouldn't mind her coming along either. Abby wasn't the sort of child who'd get under anyone's feet, and I definitely knew she'd make herself useful. I smiled to myself. Yes, I thought. She'd *love* it. The mood right now suddenly seemed one hundred per cent lighter. 'Okay, you're on,' I said grinning at them both. 'Now come on, you two, let's sort this tea.'

So we did. But once again I had no idea what I was dealing with. It was to be the calm before a very big storm.

Chapter 13

Despite my spirits being lifted by the plan we'd hatched for the following weekend, by the time Abby and I climbed into the car for the hospital visit on Sunday morning I was back in sombre mood.

Friday evening had been great in the end, Kieron having stayed for a good couple of hours, and Abby had seemed genuinely excited about being my goofy son's official helper, even to the extent of badgering him about what sort of cupcakes 'we' should bake for him, and poring over cupcake-decorating sites on the laptop.

Mike had been tickled too. 'In my day they were still British and called fairy cakes,' he pretended to huff at them. 'Dainty little things – couple of mouthfuls. And they only came in two varieties – either iced with a little silver ball in the middle, or made into butterfly tops. None of this lurid-green butter-cream nonsense and cakes the actual *size* of a cup!'

Which, of course gave Kieron an excuse to rib him mercilessly, for knowing about cakes topped with butterflies. All good family fun and all heartening for Abby, but, at the same time, you were now never far from a reminder that poor little Abby was still struggling with her demons. Sitting at the dining table when Bob was around was a clear indication. He ambled past at one point and sniffed her knee with his wet nose, and if she could have got her legs up any higher they'd have been under her chin.

'And why does she do that thing with the door frame?' Kieron had whispered as I said goodbye to him on the doorstep. He'd noticed the things with Bob too. And also the fact that it was getting worse. 'Did you see it? All that tapping her fingers on the frame before she goes into a room?'

'She can't help it, love,' I'd whispered back. 'It's all a part of the anxiety problems she has to deal with. All to do with having been separated from her mother. It's like a ritual she has to perform to keep herself calm.' I pulled the door closer behind me. She'd gone up for her bath, but she might have popped down for something. 'You might have come across it in your training, actually,' I said. 'From her symptoms, Dr Shackleton thinks she might be suffering from something called OCD.'

Which Kieron had apparently heard of, and could understand too. A need for ordering and controlling of your environment was a factor in Asperger's. Though where, in Kieron's case, it was just a part of his make-up – and something he had learned to manage – with OCD it was different. It was distressing, and obviously an escalating mental-health problem, which could be treated – and that's what Abby badly needed. To my mind, anyway, but once again I had to rein myself in.

However much that bald patch, and everything else, played on my mind, it wasn't my place to play professional here. I'd logged it all, and would now hand that responsibility over to Bridget, when she came to the house for our meeting on Thursday – where I'd urge her to get Abby to her GP. Right now, though, I was just happy that we were driving to the hospital and that Abby would have some time with Mum at last.

The weather was kinder – for the first time since we'd been there, it was sunny, rather than gloomy and raining. And, it being Sunday, and free of outpatient clinics, we didn't have to park half a mile away, either.

But that was pretty much where the positives ended.

To be fair, Sarah did look pretty washed out. She no longer had the rigid frame over her legs, I noticed, just the bulk of a plaster, so I imagined they'd dealt with whatever post-operative things they'd had to do. But she was now connected to a drip, running from the back of her hand. It might have been a painkiller, I supposed, or perhaps a drug infusion of some sort. But, as I reminded myself again, not my business.

'Poppet!' she called to Abby, as we entered the little side room. The ward, too, was quiet. No sign of Chelsea. Just a couple of visitors and, once again, I couldn't help but think surely there must be *someone*. Just someone who Abby could make a connection with, however small. Just so she didn't feel quite so alone.

'I'll leave you two to it,' I told Sarah, now I'd delivered her. 'Pop back in half an hour or so, see how you're both doing.' I had my usual clutch of gossip mags, together with one I didn't usually buy – one about baking, which had all sorts of elaborately decorated cupcakes on the cover. Might as well gen up, I'd thought, since Abby was clearly so enthused about it all; it was a great opportunity for us to do something positive together and take her mind off all the woe in her life.

And enthused she obviously was. When I returned to the pair of them, she'd told Sarah all about it.

'I hear Abby's going to be doing something for Sport Relief next weekend,' she said to me. 'With your son.'

'Yes, that's right,' I agreed. 'My sister's putting it on.' I smiled at Abby. 'We're going to be doing some baking this week, aren't we? Perhaps we could bring some cakes in for Mum next time …'

Abby nodded. 'And the nurses,' she said. 'They'd probably like some cakes, too, wouldn't they?'

I smiled. 'I've never met a nurse who wasn't grateful for a cupcake. Several cupcakes, in fact … So. Are you planning to do some reading? I've got to go and call Mike and check he's put the joint in for dinner. Do you want a bit longer? There's no real rush, really.'

Abby was perched on the bed, her mother's free arm around her. She turned to her. 'Shall I get a new book for you, Mummy? Or are you still on the last one?' She seemed to think for a moment, her expression concerned. 'Do they have anyone to read for you in here?'

Sarah shook her head. 'It's fine. I haven't felt much up to stories this past week, to be honest. But now you're here –' she glanced at me now – 'that would be *lovely*. I miss you reading to me, poppet, I really do. But, I tell you what. Why don't you go down to the little library and see if there's a book of short stories or something? That way we can read a whole one and I won't have to worry about remembering the plot for next time. That sound like a plan?'

Abby nodded happily, got down from the bed and trotted off. I was about to do likewise when Sarah beckoned that I stay.

'Is she okay?' she remarked, as soon as Abby had disappeared down the ward corridor. 'I mean, she seems bright enough, but ... well, I can't seem to get anything out of her. Not about school, what she's been up to, about how she's doing ... it's like she clams up. *Is* she doing okay at school? I worry about her constantly. And what's with all this going off to the toilet every two minutes? Three times she's been, since she got here. Has she had a tummy bug or something?'

Sarah was obviously concerned, but how much should I tell her? There was this voice in my head – it lived permanently on my shoulder – which said 'do not discuss the child with the parents – not your job'. But this was an unusual situation, wasn't it? Perhaps it would be helpful for all of us, if I shared my concerns. Perhaps she'd have some insights she could share with me about Abby. Maybe there was a background to her behaviours that could throw some useful light on how I could best manage her now. And in the light of what Abby had said to me about feeling so alone in the world, perhaps there was also someone Sarah could put me in touch with who, even if they weren't in a position to take care of her, could at least help support her, even if it was just the odd walk in the park or trip to the shops. I decided to plunge in.

'Not a bug, no,' I told Sarah. 'She has this thing about hand washing. She worries terribly about germs, as you probably already know, and it's getting to be something of a concern, I'll admit.' I went on to detail, albeit as lightly as I could, a few of the concerns we'd been having and how I'd be talking it over with her social worker later in the week, so they could take a view about whether some counselling or CBT might be in order. Sarah's expression, all the while, was growing increasingly concerned looking. But perhaps that was understandable. This was her little girl, after all. 'And I do really worry about how isolated she is,' I finished. 'I keep trying to suggest she have someone over after school or something, but it's like she doesn't have a friend in the whole world.' I frowned. 'And she feels it. Feels it keenly, I know.

'Which is why,' I went on (in for a penny, in for a pound now), 'I was wondering if there's anyone – anyone at all … some family member, or close friend – just anyone who could perhaps spare some time for her. Not take care of her – we're obviously aware of the situation in that regard. Just someone she knows well, who could give her a link to her own life, and –'

'God,' Sarah retorted, really shocking me. I had expected concern, yes, but not to be snapped at. But she was certainly snapping now. 'You just don't give up, do you?' She exhaled angrily. 'Look, she's *always* been a quiet child, *okay*? She's never much done friends. And believe me, I'm well aware of the part I've played in that. *Well* aware. So I don't need it rubbing in. But when are you people going to give this up? I've told you, there isn't *anyone*. Why d'you think I'm in this shitty bloody position?'

I blinked at the swearing. It was so sudden. And so vehement. 'I'm sorry, I –'

'There is *no one*,' she snapped over me. 'No parents, no grandparents, no knight in shining armour. What part of no one do you lot not understand? *God*. All I get is bloody social workers interrogating me!'

I didn't know what to say. I was still open-mouthed by her outburst. So I said nothing. And in the silence she seemed to gather herself a little. Perhaps most of this was what she'd wanted to say to Bridget – or whoever her own social worker was. Had she even been appointed one yet? 'Look,' she said, less stridently, perhaps seeing how shocked I looked, 'please can't you see this from *my* position? I'm laid up here, in agony half the time, and I'm constantly stressed about my baby. As I'm sure *you* would be in my shoes –'

'Of *course* I would.'

'Exactly. So you know …' Her voice was cracking now, her chin wobbling. 'I *really* can't be dealing with being told she's bloody unravelling, okay? *You're* the expert. *You're* the one who's supposed to be taking care of her, but now all I'm hearing is … *God* …' She leaned across to try and pluck a tissue from her bedside cabinet. But she couldn't reach it. So I grabbed the box and held it out to her.

'I'm sorry,' she said, snatching one out and quickly scouring her face with it. 'God, Sarah, get yourself *together here, will you?*' She looked up at me. 'I'm sorry,' she said again. 'I didn't mean to snap at you. I know it's not really your fault. It's just that I am so sick of –'

She glanced past me then. We could both hear the squeak of Abby's trainers returning.

'I'm sorry, too,' I said. 'And look, well, I'm on top of things, okay?'

Sarah noisily blew her nose. 'Ah!' she said to Abby, who had indeed returned now. 'Honestly!' she said, screwing the tissue into her palm. 'You come into hospital, and what do you get? A streaming flipping cold! Runny nose, runny eyes … Come on up, poppet.' She patted the covers. 'Let's see what you've brought to read to me, eh?'

I left them to it, but not before meeting Sarah's eye again. And feeling a profound sense of unease.

Chapter 14

'Well, well, well, Abby, it sounds like you've been a busy lady this week, then! I wish I'd come on Friday now, so I could see the finished masterpieces in all their glory!'

It was the following Thursday afternoon, and Abby was just home from school. An hour and a half earlier, Bridget had finally come for her visit, looking as brisk and efficient and on top of things as she had the last time, though with little more in her file that was useful. Her only news had been the news I'd half expected anyway – that they had drawn a blank where finding any family members was concerned, and that, given the current situation with Sarah's condition, a new permanent foster family were actively being sought. 'After all,' she'd commented, 'you and Mike are far too valuable a resource to be tied up for too long with a placement such as this one, who we should be able to slot into the mainstream so easily. We have two children right now who are in desperate need of places with experienced behaviour specialists.' She'd frowned then. 'You know how it is. We're all so stretched.'

I'd not made it obvious, but I'd really taken issue with that. To Bridget, it seemed, Mike and I were a 'resource', and Abby wasn't a desperate little girl. She was a 'placement', who could easily be 'slotted into the mainstream'. And I knew why, as well – because she was a quiet girl, and she had no 'previous' – not in terms of bad behaviour, or a history of failed placements. So, like the cutest-looking puppy in the dogs' home shop window, she should be snapped up in a moment. Job done.

It wasn't fair of me – I knew that. Bridget didn't mean it like that; she was just talking in professional jargon out of habit. But still it rankled, because it brought it home to me how easy it was for any of us to look at the packaging – in this case, a sweet, well-behaved, biddable girl – and underestimate the damage that was going on inside. And to be fair to Bridget, once I'd spent half an hour expressing the depth of my concern about Abby's OCD-like behaviour, she did have a bit of a perspective shift, and promised that before any placement was identified there would of course be a LAC review, which would be scheduled as a priority. The acronym LAC stood for 'looked after child', and it would be a review at which all Abby's needs would be discussed and any specialist requirements flagged up, including an urgent recommendation that she see her local GP. After that, as was usual, the request for suitable carers would go to panel. This was the professional body that matched potential carers with particular children. She assured me that everything possible would be done to ensure that Abby got exactly what she needed. I was grateful to know that was happening, of course, even if it felt as if it sealed her new fate – that her mother and she were to be parted. 'I still find it incredible,' I admitted, 'that Sarah has no friends to call on at a time like this, though. How do you get to be so isolated?'

Bridget had an immediate answer to that. 'By having to keep your circumstances quiet over a very long period.'

'Yes, but that completely? What about old friends? I don't know – from her antenatal group or something? And neighbours – where are they? Can people really cut themselves off so much? But she was adamant. Absolutely adamant, when I asked her at the weekend.'

Bridget's ears seemed to prick up when I said this. 'Oh,' she said. 'I bet she'll have *loved* that. She's already sick of us lot badgering her, that's been pretty clear.'

'Tell me about it,' I said, wincing at the memory, which still bothered me. 'I think I got both barrels.'

'But I can't say I'm surprised,' Bridget said, her tone subtly different now. She slid a bookmark into her journal. She'd made plenty of notes, at least. Now all she had to do was act on them. And if not, I'd take Abby to my own flipping GP. 'You know, Casey,' she went on, placing her pen on the dining table, 'don't take offence or anything, but you know you really don't want to be getting involved in Sarah's family circumstances. She's already made it clear to us how the land lies in that respect, as you know.'

Casey Watson

I felt myself begin to bridle. 'I know that,' I said. 'And I wasn't interrogating her on her family tree, Bridget, simply asking her if there was friend who could support Abby, that's all.'

'Yes, I *do* know,' she said, not quite meeting my eye. 'But there are some things that, well … are really for *us* to deal with. You have enough on your plate –' Now she did meet my eye, and smiled at me. 'Looking after little Abby. Doing your *own* job …'

The rest was something of a blur, I was so angry. Where had *that* come from? Christ, was it my week for being got at, or what?

Then Abby's taxi home from school pulled up, a life-saving ten minutes later. I actually thought it was silly, that she was still being taken there and back by cab. Yes, it was a long drive for me, but what a lonely business that must be for her, and I didn't understand why it was necessary. Something I should bring up, though perhaps not today. But I couldn't have been happier to see it at that moment, for sure.

And now all three of us were in the kitchen, having a cup of tea and some biscuits, and Abby (having washed her hands twice already – which I drew attention to, and Bridget duly noted) was showing Bridget all the cup-cake designs that, in theory, were going to be a reality by this time tomorrow.

And beautiful they all would be as well, we all agreed, but I was counting the minutes till I could see Bridget out. How dare she speak to me like that? How dare she!

* * *

'Can you believe it?' I ranted at Mike as soon as he got home from work. I'd been so cross that, once we'd finished making several batches of coloured icing, ready for finishing off with Abby tomorrow, I embarked on a full-on clean-up in the kitchen. Much as I understood that Abby's passion for cleaning was a bad thing, for me it was the best way I knew to relieve stress: stuff the cupcakeathon, what I needed was a good, full-on scrubathon, and, despite it being the opposite of what Dr Shackleton had suggested, today I let her don her marigolds and scrub along with me.

'Calm down, love,' Mike said, as he changed out of his work gear. I'd left Abby in the kitchen zapping the skirting boards with my germ spray, and had followed him straight upstairs. 'She's just being officious – you've got to admit, she always did look officious – and you know what social services are like with all their who-must-do-what stuff. Take no notice.'

'I was being warned off, is what was happening there,' I persisted. 'The cheek of it! Like it's such a terrible thing to ask someone a perfectly reasonable question! Just what's so bad about having a conversation about how best a mother might help her own flipping child?!'

'But it's not about what you asked her. It's the fact *that* you asked her. And … I don't know … maybe they know something about her that you don't. Maybe she's already told them to back off – sounds like she might well have done that, doesn't it? And now Bridget's worried they'll get it in the neck all over again. Or that relations will break down, and things will get even more difficult. Who knows?'

I had to concede that Mike was right. He invariably was. And I knew I sometimes got my knickers in a twist about being on the periphery of all the important decisions, despite being the one who was closest to the child. It had happened to me before, and I knew – when I was thinking rationally, at least – that it was just the nature of the job of fostering. Yes, I was closest to the child, but the child was in the care of social services and there were sound reasons why, charged with responsibility for that child's welfare, it was social services that had to make sure all the paperwork was correct. After all, social services were where the buck stopped.

When I came back downstairs to start on tea, Abby was on her hands and knees in the kitchen, scrubbing away at the place where the wall met the floor, using what looked like a toothbrush. She looked up as I came in.

'Oh,' she said, waving it at me. I'd been right. It *was* a toothbrush. 'I hope this is all right. I found it in your box under the sink, so I thought it must be your brush for getting into all the little corners.'

I had never actually scrubbed out a little corner with a toothbrush – even my cleaning mania didn't extend that far. It was actually what I used to scrub the mildew out of the detergent dispenser in the washing machine, but even as I thought it I didn't bother correcting her. Perhaps there was little to choose between the two things anyway.

'That's fine,' I said, 'but, come on, enough for one day, Cinderella. Time to get ourselves straight and get the tea show on the road, eh?'

She stood up then, and went over to the sink to rinse the toothbrush. She had a peaceful look about her. What a complicated child she was. 'Are you looking forward to Saturday?' I asked her as I cleared the worktop. 'I know my sister's looking forward to meeting you. And you know my niece, Chloe, will be there. She's fourteen. You'll like her. She's a big *Glee* fan as well.'

'I can't wait,' Abby answered. And I was pretty sure she meant it.

Attachment theory is one of those subjects that can be really, really interesting, or really, really dull, depending on whom it is who's explaining it. Halfway into our introductory lecture, which was taking place in one of those out-of-the-way centres that local councils maintain just for the purpose, the fact that I was nodding off didn't augur well for the remaining few hours.

Not that I wasn't interested. Attachment theory – first described by the psychologist John Bowlby – was perhaps the single most common thread that ran through everything we did as foster carers. So many ills of the world could perhaps be attributed to little children not having been able to form a strong attachment to their mums (or, to use the parlance, 'primary caregivers').

Almost every child we cared for had had some sort of issue in this regard, so it was a useful – perhaps necessary

– part of our continuing training that we understood how these essential human attachments worked.

This had obviously not been the case for Abby, however, and it was to her that my mind kept straying. Though with the distraction of the 'cupcakeathon' she'd been reasonably okay this week, it was still pretty tough, because yet again it had been decided that with Sarah's current treatment being so intense it would be best if they continued on just phone calls during the week nights, and a visit on the Sunday, as before. I had my own thoughts about that – were they stretching the gap between visits in order to start preparing her for what was to come? No one had said anything to me, but it felt that way. I was also still smarting at being ticked off by Bridget for overstepping the boundaries of 'my position' in wanting to try and do my best for Abby. And though I knew Mike was right in what he'd said about that, I still couldn't help but feel huffy about it, which was making my mind stray a little.

I also couldn't help thinking about what was going to become of her. All the previous kids we'd fostered had been in such a bad place when they'd come to us that whatever happened to them – and good outcomes were by no means guaranteed for them – we were at least working on the premise that, however things turned out for them, it was unlikely to be worse than where they'd come from. They'd come from hellish lives – lives of neglect, abuse and heart-break – and we were a step on the road to them reclaiming their childhoods, nurtured and supported, if not by their own parents, then by people who really cared about what happened to them, in most cases, for the first time in their lives.

This was not true – and wouldn't be true – of Abby. Yes, if they found a caring foster home, she perhaps would reclaim her childhood, and, all being well, her mother's illness would be controlled sufficiently that she would have many years yet in which to be a positive influence in her daughter's life. But however socially and morally unacceptable Abby's lifestyle had been, it was Abby's home and Abby's life and she'd clearly always felt safe and loved there. There was no lack of attachment between mother and daughter, so to be wrenched apart permanently would break both their hearts. What hope for Abby's mental demons then?

We were let out eventually, and, in the end, it had been quite interesting. Though by the time I arrived at my sister's café I was dying for a cup of tea. What was it about sitting listening that made you feel so sluggish? And, come to think of it, so parched?

I'd not had a chance to stop by at Donna's place since Abby had been with us, and was pleased to see how well my little sis was evidently doing. Mid-afternoon on an overcast March Saturday was always going to be a good bet for a café off a high street, but I could tell the place – still busy – had been buzzing all day. And our cupcake contribution had gone down a storm.

'They've all gone!' Abby said triumphantly as I got to her. She was stationed in the little room out the back of the café, counting out a big tub of coins with Chloe, and I made a mental note to check with Donna if she and her brother would be around to come along to Jackson and Abby's rearranged birthday party. Kieron, meanwhile, was stationed at the state-of-the-art coffee machine they'd installed – and of which I approved unreservedly.

'Come on,' said Donna, as Kieron presented me with one of the café's finest, 'let's leave the girls to it and go out front. There's a table free in the window. You hungry?'

'Famished,' I told her. 'I skipped the buffet to drive back here. Which was no hardship, believe me. Wall-to-wall flipping sausage rolls and egg mayo sandwiches. Ugh. Took me straight back to when we were kids. So if you've got something nicer …'

'You bet,' she said. 'So go grab the table, while I get us a couple of decent sandwiches. If I don't sit down soon I shall fall down.'

It was always good to catch up with my sister. Even though there were four years between us, as youngsters we'd been inseparable. I'd really missed her when she'd been living across the water, on the Emerald Isle. 'And what a sweetie Abby is,' Donna said. 'She's a darling. Massive crush on your Kieron, of course – but that's understandable, as he has the family good looks …' This was a standing joke. We were all short. Kieron was six foot two. We were all dark – Donna and I black-haired – Kieron was blond. He was the spit of his father, end of. 'Anyway,' Donna went on, through a mouthful of sandwich, 'she's not what I was expecting, at all.' I'd filled Donna in a little about Abby's situation and her problems, and how she shouldn't worry too much about her hand-washing and her tics. 'She's been a treasure, she has. Worked like a little Trojan all morning. Though we did give her a lunch break, you'll be pleased to know – Riley and the kids came in with Mike and they took her off to McDonald's.' Donna laughed. 'Seems she preferred that to the idea of one of our posh designer sandwiches.'

'Which *are* exceedingly posh,' I agreed, having now finished the first half of mine.

'Hey, sis, what you expect? You're in the posh part of town now. No plastic ham and marge round this manor!'

I could see Abby from where we were sitting, busy making little piles of coins with Chloe. 5ps and 2ps and 20ps, in neat stacks. And it took me back to when my own two were her age, and school fêtes, and how much fun they used to have when I was on the parent–teacher association, when they'd help on the stalls and with the displays and the setting up, and how we'd all sit round afterwards – teachers and parents and kids alike – doing exactly the same thing. It was an education itself, raising money for charity. I presumed Abby had no such sense of community in her school, because her mum had so little to do with it herself.

Donna followed my gaze. 'So what's going to happen to her now, then? She'll be fostered permanently? Poor thing. What a rubbish hand to have been dealt, eh?'

'You're telling me,' I agreed. 'But I don't think there's any other option.'

'But at least there are some good people out there – *that's* what you need to remember. And let's not forget, compared with some of the kids you've had, things aren't so bad for her. Look at Justin, for one. At least she's got a mum who loves her. And fingers crossed, that's not going to change. And, as I always say, you have love, you have almost all you need in life. And there endeth the homily. Another coffee?'

I smiled. Trust my sister to put a positive spin on things. We were two peas in a pod, too. 'Is the Pope Catholic?' I asked her. She gestured to Kieron to rustle up two more.

'Oh, and by the way,' she said, 'your boy there tells me Abby's asked if she can come and help again next time he's in. I said I'd have to check with you, because I don't know what the rules are with your foster kids. I mean, not to work, obviously, but if she wants to, and you think she'd get something out of it, I've no objections if she wants to come down for an hour or two with him here and there. She can write my price tickets for me, decorate the menus or whatever. She just *loved* getting her hands on my blackboard and my liquid-chalk marker pens. Of course, she might just want to gaze adoringly at young Adonis there … ah! Here you are, Kieron. Best barista in the western world, bar none!'

I sipped my second coffee and felt my own pleasing glow of positivity. Assuming you weren't God, then you obviously couldn't perform miracles, but while Abby was with us we could at least do our best for her. And how lovely it would be for her to broaden her horizons that little bit. A couple of hours here and there probably meant nothing to the average person, but to a child held virtual prisoner by the need to care for her sick mother a couple of hours of doing anything that took her out of home and drudgery were definitely a couple of hours well spent.

And Kieron was police checked, so there was no problem if he was with her. Bless my sister. 'Thank you. I'm sure she'd love that,' I told her.

Chapter 15

Heading back to the hospital on the following morning, Abby was full of her exploits of the previous day. She'd clearly got a lot out of it and, though I was still playing hawk eye as far as her hand-washing and switch-flicking and hair-pulling were concerned, I felt the same sense of optimism as I had the previous afternoon. Maybe Donna had put something in my coffee.

My spirits dampened just a little when we arrived at the hospital. Not a lot, but there's something I've never quite liked about hospitals on a weekend. I think it's the lack of activity. There's no outpatient clinics, no hustle and bustle, no operations going on, no ward rounds or physiotherapists to fill the wards and corridors – just the stark reality of sick people in beds.

Not that I intended spending too much time by Sarah's bed. After last week's little outburst and Bridget's subsequent pointed comments, I'd decided to keep well away from any conversations about Abby. If Sarah asked me anything then I would of course answer her. But my main priority was simply to deliver Abby to her bedside, then bugger off to a seat by the vending machines. I might even explore further – there'd be a restaurant somewhere, wouldn't there? Perhaps I'd go and find it, and read my stash of mags there – not forgetting to once again call Mike with the instructions about the roast. But not yet – he'd already been picked up by Riley's David before we'd left, as he was going to help him erect a garden shed.

And it was no bother, slinking away, because Sarah, still with her drip attached, didn't seem interested in talking to me either. Abby was so full of her cake-decorating skills – we'd saved a little box of cupcakes for Sarah and the nurses – that I was superfluous from the off. Which was just fine by me.

Indeed, the only words we exchanged were when I returned to collect Abby.

'Sounds like Abby's having a wonderful weekend,' Sarah commented, while Abby repacked her backpack. She'd also taken along some photos of the charity event to show her mum. Kieron had uploaded them on Facebook so we could print some off to show her. 'And popping back on Tuesday, I hear –'

'I told you, Mum. I'm going to be Kieron's official helper,' Abby corrected her. 'And Donna said I can be in charge of doing the blackboard again as well.'

'She's a very talented calligrapher,' I chipped in. 'Seriously. Really good.'

'She is indeed,' Sarah said, nodding, 'and it's very kind of your son – and your sister – to take an interest in Abby. I appreciate it.'

'Don't mention it,' I said. 'She's no trouble at all. Quite the opposite, in fact –'

'I've been indips-indis-pensable,' Abby said. 'Donna said so. She said I was the best little grafter she ever saw.'

Which made me smile. It was obviously a matter of great pride to Abby. Being indispensable had been a burden she had carried for so long that needing to be so was probably now in her DNA. Which was fine, just as long as it was channelled in a *good* way so that, though she felt it, she didn't need to actually *be* it. And I had a hunch Sarah knew that, as well.

As planned, Kieron came round to pick Abby up the following Tuesday afternoon, and took her off to Truly Scrumptious for a couple of hours before tea. And, once again, on their return I sensed a new lightness in Abby. And though I worried that perhaps it was all just feeding into her compulsions (all that necessary hand washing, and cleaning, and donning of her precious pinny) I reminded myself that it wasn't really for me to tackle things. I was still disrupting her rituals as much as possible while I was around her at home, but something told me anyway that she was all the better for a change of scenery and focus. It was a distraction and I felt sure it was doing her good.

And Donna was spot on – Abby had definitely developed something of a crush on Kieron, and I thought again of the father figure she'd evidently never had. It was sweet to see, and, again, I felt it was another positive. Kieron naturally chose to do things that worked well with her psyche, and as they told me how they'd redesigned the back wall behind the counter I could see the same zeal for order in both their eyes, imagining the pair of them pinning up price lists with a set square and lining up everything to the nearest millimetre.

'Oh, and we're coming to tea Thursday,' Kieron said before he left. 'Me and Lauren. I've promised Abs here that we'll take her down to the woods before tea. There should be frogspawn there now, hopefully, so I said we could collect some for her school project in a couple of weeks. That's okay, isn't it?'

'You mean the tea?' I said, privately touched by this gesture. I didn't even *know* about the school project. 'Or the filling my house with tadpoles?' I continued. 'Just so I'm clear …' I said, grinning at the pair of them. 'Of course, love. That's *fine*. Maybe Levi could join you. He'd love that –'

I watched Abby's face cloud over and her shoulders tense up. I could read her thoughts too: *But it's dangerous in the woods. He might get hurt. And I won't be able to relax …* It was probably half-subconscious, but it was as clear as the stream water. 'Actually, there's a thought. I think Riley has something on with the kids. No matter.' And, as if pushed, Abby's shoulders went back down again. So easy to forget, I thought, how much this kid needed one simple thing – to not feel responsible for anyone but herself – indips-indispensable or otherwise.

'We'd better dig that old tank out, then, hadn't we?' I said.

But the week wasn't done with surprising either me or the frogspawn. With Wednesday came unexpected news from my sister. News that was to unleash a great deal more chaos in my little pond than any amount of tadpoles could ever do.

'You got five minutes,' Donna asked me, 'for a quick chinwag, by any chance?' It was ten in the morning, and with Abby safely in school for the day, I was just finishing up my chores before heading off to Riley's. Once again the party was back on the agenda, and I was keen to make it a good one, for Abby's sake as much as Jackson's. I was determined that her tenth birthday was not going to go unremarked.

'Sure, 'I said. 'How's things? How did things go with Abby? Did you give her free rein with your chalk pens again?'

'It's Abby I'm calling about, as it happens,' said Donna. 'And what we were talking about over the weekend.'

I sat down on the stairs – my usual station when on the phone. 'As in?'

'As in what you were saying about there being no family around.'

Had Abby said something to Donna? Or maybe to Kieron, perhaps? 'And?'

'And there might be,' Donna said. 'Well, in theory, at any rate. You know when she was in here yesterday? Well, she was behind the counter, putting back all the menus into their holders – did a great job, by the way. We are now seriously floralled up down here ... Anyway, I've got this regular, Mrs Shelley. Sweetheart, she is. Little old lady. Comes in at least twice a week. And she starts chatting to Abby, and I'm kind of earwigging, as you do. And it turns out they know each other. They used to be neighbours.'

'Really?' I felt my ears pricking up now.

'Indeed. So she's asking Abby how she is, and how "poor Mum" is – I picked up on that one straight away – and Abby's explaining that her mum's in hospital and that Abby herself is currently staying in a "care home" – thought that might make you smile, sis! – so I get Mrs Shelley her tea and cake and take it over to her table, and then I scoot back to Abby and she tells me that they used to live on the same street, and how nice Mrs Shelley was and how she'd felt so sad when they'd had to move.'

'And there's more, right?'

'Oh, yes. I obviously didn't say any more to Abby, but when she and Kieron had gone – Mrs Shelley had come in just before they were going, handily – I decided, in light of what you'd said about the circumstances, to see if Mrs Shelley could tell me any more. And indeed she could ...'

I waited. And I waited. 'Go on, then!'

'Shh ... I'm just building the suspense! Anyway, Mrs Shelley was most enlightening. I obviously didn't say too much to her – only corroborated what Abby had already told her, and confirmed that her mum was pretty ill and so on. And that right now it was looking unlikely that she'd be able to go home with Abby, as now Pandora was out of the box, so to speak, in terms of how they'd been living, it wasn't a situation they could return to. And Mrs Shelley was like "Oh, I know. I so felt for that little girl!" She'd see her in the post office every week, apparently, paying the rent, and getting tokens for their gas and electricity meters, and she'd see her struggling to put the bins out – this was from quite an early age, apparently – and how she'd never accept any help from her or anything.

'In fact she told me that she'd been seriously close to calling social services, and it was only for fear of Abby being taken into care that she hadn't – mainly because she liked Sarah and that, while she knew she had health issues, she just kept hoping it would turn around, and she'd get better. And because of Abby, too, she said. Because how could there be anything *so* wrong, when she was always such a nice, polite little girl? And that's pretty much it. She just couldn't bring herself to do it.'

'I can understand that.'

'Ah, but then came the main thing. She suddenly goes to me, "But what about Sarah's sister? Couldn't someone get in touch with her, perhaps?"'

'*Wow.*'

'And that's pretty much all I know. Oh, and that she thinks her name might have been Vicky. And that she was around quite a lot until Abby was two or three. And then she didn't see her again. I suppose it's possible she might have died, of course.'

'But Sarah would have said so. If she was dead, Sarah would have said so, surely. But I've never even *heard* of the existence of a sister. Which is interesting.'

'Isn't it? Anyway, I thought you'd like to know. She'll be back in again – Mrs Shelley, that is – so do you want me to get her number? I'm sure she'd talk to you. She said she'd be happy to do anything she could.'

'No, no. No, don't bother her,' I said. 'I'll have a think.' *And run this past John*, I decided. *See what he says*. Well, well, well, I thought. Well, well, well.

I called John the very minute I put the phone down on Donna. There was no way I was going to mention it to Bridget. Not without running it by John first. I felt sure she'd just use it as another stick to beat me with, cite some reason why my coming by this information was against some important protocol. Not that it was necessarily going to be helpful anyway. And if this sister existed, why hadn't those distant cousins mentioned it? Or if they had, why hadn't anyone picked up on it?

Or perhaps they had, and it had already proved to be a cul-de-sac. Perhaps that was one of the reasons why Sarah had been so irritable when I'd seen her. But it didn't figure. If there'd been a sister, and she'd been ruled out, surely I'd have known that? Bridget would have said, 'The cousins are out of the picture, *and so is the sister.*' Nope, as far as social services went, this sister clearly didn't even exist. Of that I was sure. But the question was, why?

John's office phone rang for so long that I nearly disconnected and called his mobile. But I was glad I didn't because when the answerphone finally kicked in it informed me of something I knew but had forgotten – that John was off having a much-needed two weeks of doing nothing, with his wife, for their twenty-fifth wedding anniversary, and wouldn't be back for a fortnight.

I put the phone down again. There was no way I was going to call him on holiday. He had enough on his plate already, running the agency. No, I'd let him have his holiday. This was hardly life and death. But still I rejected the idea of calling Bridget. I'd wait for Mike to get home and see what he thought about it. And in the meantime get to Riley's and put it right out of my mind.

'And that's where it should stay. At least till John gets back from holiday.' Mike was in no doubt about it. I'd filled him in, once again, as soon as he got home, following him around the house as he changed out of his work clothes.

'Do nothing?'

'Do nothing. There'll be a reason this woman's not been mentioned. She could be a monster. Who knows? Or an old lag. Or a prostitute. There are a million families with skeletons – and a million black sheep out there. You and I, of all people, should know that. Besides, you know how mad you are about Bridget citing protocol; it's not your place to be digging up worms about this woman, is it?'

'You mean opening a can of them –'

Mike tutted. 'Okay, Mrs Clever-clogs. Whatever. But you get my point. It's not your business, and it might make things worse.'

'Can they *get* any worse? For Abby? Come on ... Not to mention Sarah.'

'Oh, yes,' said Mike, signalling that this really was the end of it. 'There's a reason why people are told to count their blessings. There's *always* scope for things to get worse.'

Chapter 16

But in the end, events overtook me. Well, not overtook me, exactly, just sidled up alongside me, causing my firm resolution – which was to leave things, at least till after John's second honeymoon – to veer so spectacularly off the road.

The rest of the week had been uneventful. Abby didn't mention Mrs Shelley in the café – why would she? She was ten and this was just an old neighbour from her past. She was much more fixated on the here and now of her life, which was falling into a routine which seemed to be at least manageable. I was keeping a particularly close eye on her scalp, of course. I would draw attention to it every time her hand went to her temple, and though she would deal with that by having to perform some other ritual – say, tapping the door frame, or patting the closest light switch – those felt the lesser of two evils and that was good enough for now. There was the constant stress, of course, about having to be near a hot tap and a supply of liquid soap – but with these now being something I expected (and understanding the reasons) I wasn't fretting about them as much as before. Bridget had also emailed to say they'd set a date for the LAC review, and promised to follow up on a GP visit, so I knew some support would now be forthcoming for Abby. Which was one less thing to feel anxious about too.

'Thursday, too, came and went without incident – though also without tadpoles. Kieron had got himself an unexpected gig, which meant some money, and though he told me he'd turn it down, both Lauren and I were adamant he didn't; it was a kind gesture, and of course Abby would be disappointed, but he had to be practical about things. Lauren was happy to take Abby to the woods, as was I, but when it came to it the rain was hammering down that day anyway, and Abby didn't seem in the least concerned about forgoing it. 'I mean, I'll go if Lauren really, really wants to,' she'd confided to me when she got in from school. 'But it'll be awfully muddy, won't it?' She'd wrinkled her nose up delicately. 'And we might slip over and that wouldn't be very nice …'

Suppressing a smile at her wonderful talent for understatement, I assured her that Lauren wouldn't mind. I had half a hunch that it wasn't just about germs in this case, either. She wanted Kieron there. Which was absolutely fine.

And now it was Sunday again, and we were back at the hospital, and, once again, the mysterious sister was back on my mind. Not that I had any intention of mentioning her. As before my only plan was to deliver Abby safely, let them have forty-five minutes, then take her back home. It was Abby who pulled the lid open on Pandora's Box this time.

'Guess who I saw last week?' she told her mother as I approached, having done the coffee, done the gossip mags and was now fully conversant with which key looks were 'on-trend' for the coming summer.

'Erm ...' said Sarah, who'd seemed in brighter spirits than the last time I'd seen her. I had no idea what was happening with her trial or her medication, and, my fingers already singed, I was not about to ask. 'Father Christmas?'

'NO, silly!'

'The Easter bunny?'

'Too early!'

'The Scarlet Pimpernel?'

'Who's the Scarlet Pimpernel? I've never even heard of the Scarlet Pimpernel.'

'Because he's the Scarlet Pimpernel – and he likes to lie low. They seek him here, they seek him there ...'

Abby shook her head. 'Definitely not him, then.'

'Go on, then,' said Sarah, grinning. 'I can't guess.'

'Mrs Shelley. When I was working in Casey's sister's café with Kieron, on Tuesday. I meant to tell you on the phone, but I forgot.'

The grin vanished. Sarah's eyes flicked from mine and back to Abby's. I'd been clutching my carrier bag of magazines so tightly that I could feel the plastic cutting into my fingers. I slid my own gaze to the window, and tried to look as if I was miles away.

'Did you, now?' said Sarah. 'And how is she?'

Abby shrugged. 'Oh, she's fine. She said to send her love. I told her you were in hospital having a relapse.'

Sarah didn't seem to know what to say to that. There was a short but intense silence, which grew more uncomfortable by the second. And spoke volumes. Was almost deafening, in fact. Then Abby spoke again. 'She goes into Casey's sister's café every week, you know. So I told her next time I'm working there I'll tell her which ward you're on. I couldn't remember the name of it, but I've written it on my list now, so I don't forget it for next time. I think she wants to send you a card. Or she might want to come and visit you …'

'*Visit* me?' Sarah looked stricken. 'Oh, I don't think she'll want to do that.'

I could feel her eyes on me again now. 'Oh, I think she would,' said Abby. 'I told her you don't have any visitors except me. So when she next comes in –'

'Abby, you know, I'm really not sure I'm up to having visitors. Apart from you, of course,' she added quickly. 'And Mrs Shelley … well, she's quite elderly, and it's such a long way …'

She seemed to think for a moment, clearly feeling harried by Abby's innocent insistence. 'Actually, could you do me a favour, poppet, and fill my water jug up for me before you go? You know where the drinking water tap is, don't you? Or just go and find one of the nurses. They'll do it …'

'Okay,' said Abby, trotting round to the other side of the bed to fetch it. It was three-quarters full, but she didn't question it. It had probably been sitting there a while, so she would have wanted to change it anyway. I followed Sarah's eyes as she watched her daughter take the jug away.

She turned straight to me. 'You know,' she said, 'I'm really not sure I'm happy about Abby working in your family business.'

'She's not *working* at my sister's place,' I corrected. 'She's just been down there on two occasions with my son. Once to help with a charity event, which, as you know, she really enjoyed. And then to do some colouring and cutting out after school. Because she *asked* if she could. It's hardly –'

'Even so, I'd rather she didn't do it any more.'

And that was the thing, really. If she'd left it at that, then *I'd* have left it too. After all, how could I not have? She'd made a request, and I was happy to comply with it. Well, not happy exactly – because I knew how disappointed Abby would be. But not so unhappy that I'd put myself in a difficult situation with Sarah. Yes I was *in loco parentis*, but I was also a pragmatist. And Sarah was a sick woman. And relations were strained enough already.

But she didn't leave it. I'd already nodded my acquiescence, but evidently she couldn't stop herself. 'And I don't want to see that Mrs Shelley, either. So if she comes in again and starts asking after me, I'd be grateful if you'd respect my privacy. She's a nosey old bat and she's no business talking to Abby. She shouldn't be listening to anything she says.'

It was probably that – the fact that she'd called her a nosey old bat – that meant I couldn't stop myself. There was just no call for it. I knew I had to make allowances for the desperate nature of her situation, but there was just no call for it. It was unkind. So before I could stop myself, I spoke.

'Of course,' I said. 'Of course. I wouldn't *dream* of doing otherwise. Only she said you had a sister and –'

'Rubbish!' Sarah was suddenly totally galvanised. 'That's exactly what I mean. She's talking *rubbish*!'

I noticed her hands had begun to shake and could see that Abby was returning. 'Look,' I said. 'The last thing I want to do is upset you. Just forget I ever said that. This is really none of my business. There are clearly things I don't know here, and it's not for me to get involved … just forget it, okay? Just forget it.'

Of course, forgetting it, for me, was an entirely different matter. With the atmosphere now as thick as Mike's legendary beef gravy, I wanted nothing more than to bundle Abby back out and away from the hospital as quickly as I could. Abby herself, thankfully, was oblivious, and though I had to pull her up half a dozen times about her hair on the journey, by the time we'd hit the motorway she'd dropped off to sleep, leaving me with my maelstrom of thoughts.

I had clearly touched a nerve, and a particularly raw one, and, once again, I couldn't help but speculate about the nature of the circumstances that had caused such a reaction at the mention of the sister's name. But along with the musing there was an undercurrent tugging beneath the surface; I had overstepped the mark again, wellied in where

I shouldn't. And, as soon as I was able, I would have to tell John.

But in the meantime I knew that the best thing I could do was to try to put the whole thing out of my mind.

Which was easier said than done. When I got home and confessed to Mike, he simply rolled his eyes and called me a klutz (for which I was grateful – it helped put it in perspective, which was probably what I needed), but I still had the small matter of Abby. Donna had agreed she could go in with Kieron again after school on the Tuesday, and that if she wanted to she could help her create a new weekly special for the children's menu – about which Abby had been thinking from the moment she'd been told.

She'd been poring over my recipe books all week and when she came home from school on Monday she even sat down and compiled an inventory of E numbers that she needed to check wouldn't be in any of the ingredients. I did find myself smiling – a career in health and safety wouldn't be a bad choice for her – but at the same time I was still agonising about what to say to her. I clearly couldn't let her go, even though part of me was saying 'sod it', but I also knew it wouldn't be helpful to tell her why. A white lie, I decided. I would just tell her something had come up, last minute. I didn't know what, yet, but I knew I'd come up with something. And once I'd done that I'd already planned how I'd distract her. I'd whisk her round to Riley's so we could sit down and thrash out the details of Jackson's – and her – upcoming party.

I sighed to myself as I packed Abby off to school on Tuesday morning, and felt terrible when she told me how excited she was about Kieron picking her up to 'go to work'. It didn't matter how much I told myself it wasn't the end of the world; I had the feeling that there was a cloud permanently sitting on my shoulder. No, I didn't make Mrs Shelley walk into the café, did I? And, no, I didn't ask her to recognise Abby, did I? And, no, I didn't ask Abby to bring it up with Sarah, either. Everything that had happened was outside of my control. All I did was mention something that Sarah *already knew*, which was hardly a criminal offence. But no matter how much I told myself I'd really done nothing wrong, I still felt an overriding need to 'confess'. But with John not back till the weekend I would have to wait. It was going to feel like a long, stressful week.

The phone rang just as I was pulling a pair of sponge cakes from the oven. It was just before lunchtime, and I'd made two large rectangular slabs, which were going to provide the raw materials to make Jupiter, Pontypandy fire service's fire engine. Jackson was too small to have much input on party theming, but Levi was clear – Fireman Sam would be the favourite, which was absolutely fine by me and Riley. Fine by Riley, because she was very creative – definitely the artist in the family – and fine by me because I was an old hand at fire engines: I'd already made a Fireman Sam birthday cake. Kieron had had one for his third birthday.

I was in a sentimental mood that morning, busy counting my blessings, thinking how lucky I was to be so involved in my children's lives, to be counted on, included, so immersed in my grandchildren. I was one lucky nanna, and I knew it. I was also otherwise engaged, transferring the heavy tins from oven to cooling racks, so by the time I'd whipped my oven gloves off and run into the hall the answerphone had already kicked in.

'Sorry,' I heard Mike's posh telephone voice telling the caller. 'We can't get to the phone at the moment, so please –'

I snatched the phone up. 'Hello?'

'Ah, Casey,' a voice said. A voice I knew very well.

'John? Oh! What are you doing calling me? Aren't you still on holiday?'

'I am,' he said, slowly. 'In theory.'

There was no rancour in his tone, but I didn't miss his heavy sigh. I felt my stomach knot, and waited for whatever bad thing he was going to say. He got straight to the point. And I wasn't wrong about it being a bad thing. 'Casey, we've got something of a situation.'

I felt a massive rush of guilt. So he'd been called while on his holiday. So whatever it was, it must be pretty serious.

'What sort of situation?' I asked him.

'A situation involving you. Look – God, I feel dreadful having to talk to you about this over the phone Casey, believe me –'

'Not as dreadful as I feel.'

He sighed again. 'Look, there's no point me trying to sugar this pill for you. And I wouldn't insult your intelligence by trying to do so in any case. You know how things work. There's been a complaint made against you, Casey. An official complaint, in writing, to Bridget – well, to social services, more accurately – by Abby's mother.'

I felt cold. Nothing like this had ever happened to me before, and I felt stunned, out of balance. 'For what?' My mouth had gone dry.

'Brace yourself. Three things.'

'Three? God, there's a *list*?'

'I'm afraid so. As I said, brace yourself. First, meddling in her private business. Apparently – and you can take my verbal quote marks as read, Casey, you know that – you've been grilling the hospital staff for information about her medical condition –'

I wanted to roar my denial at John, but reined myself in. *Just hear the charges first, Casey.* I licked my parched lips. 'And?'

'Causing her daughter psychological damage – causing all these "sudden" OCD symptoms. She makes mention of a bald patch … We'll come back to that …'

'And?'

'And, let me see. Yes – "using her daughter – a minor – as cheap labour in the family business".'

Now I could barely contain myself. Yet I was so appalled that I didn't know where to start.

'Casey?' John said. 'Casey, you still there?'

'Yes, I'm here, John.' I forced my mind to pull itself together. 'Right,' I said, sucking in a lungful of air. 'Firstly, I haven't "grilled" any member of Sarah's medical staff. I've barely communicated with a single nurse! Oh, unless you want to count taking in a few of Abby's cupcakes – does that count as bribery, perhaps? *Jesus*! And the only in-depth conversation I've had with anyone at that hospital was with Sarah's occupational therapist. Chelsea, her name is. Who basically sat down with me and gabbled on about all sorts of things – before I could stop her, I might add – which she clearly thought I already knew. About which, I might add, I put her straight. Secondly – actually, don't get me started on "secondly". I cannot BELIEVE she could say that! After all the years of … no …' I took another breath. 'Let's not even go there. It's just too bloody ridiculous. And as for "thirdly", well, frankly, how dare she? How DARE she!' I could feel anger rising inside me like an internal tsunami. It was so preposterous, so disgraceful, such a wicked distortion of what had happened. But as the tidal wave of fury welled up in my throat, another thought cut in. John was just the messenger. And John was still on holiday. I had no right to rant at him. I took a third breath, and then cleared my throat.

'I'm sorry, John. Let me gather myself for a moment.'

'Absolutely, Casey. This has obviously come as some-thing of a shock. And, look, you know where I stand. I am one hundred per cent behind you. Whatever accusations she's made.'

I had another thought. John didn't know about the sister. *No one* knew about the sister. And that was key. 'John, there's something you need to know about all this. I think there's a *reason* for all this. No. I KNOW there's a reason for all this.'

I told him everything I knew: what Donna had relayed about Mrs Shelley, in the café; what had happened at the hospital when Abby had mentioned her name; how Sarah had told me Abby was not allowed to go down there and 'work' any more. 'She used the term then,' I said to John. 'And I was pretty bloody peeved, I can tell you. And then she just couldn't leave it ... I don't know what the history is, John, but there's something she's keeping from us ... There's definitely something. I mean, why would you say you didn't have a sister if you had?'

'Perhaps she's dead.'

'So same question, surely? And Bridget doesn't know this. I'd already decided it probably wasn't for me to mention it. I was going to ring you when you came back, and tell you first. Let you handle it. I was already a bit twitched about talking to Bridget ...'

'And you can imagine how twitched *she* is, right now.'

Another wave began to well in me, but this time it was different. This time it was less a wave than a heavy, sicky feeling. An official complaint. Which would need investigating, however trumped up and vindictive it was. Oh, God. What would happen now? Once again, with some effort, I tried to keep myself together. 'So what's the next step?' I asked John, feeling myself failing, even so. 'God, I'm so sorry, John. I mean it. I am so, so sorry. I mean, I categorically deny everything she's accused me of, but I'm so sorry you've had all this dumped on you. I should have just let them get on with it. I've clearly rattled Sarah's cage. I should have trusted my instincts. God, I *knew* she

had it in for me. The only thing I can't figure out is
– *why*?'

'I don't think it's you, Casey. As you say, this seems to be
all about her, from what you've said. But in answer to your
question, there's a process that we've now got to go
through. A supervision meeting, in the first instance.'

'Oh, God. That sounds damning.'

'Try not to think of it in those terms. I know you don't
need any such thing. You and Mike are my shining stars.
Remember that. Honestly, Casey, please don't worry
about it. But yes, that's what'll happen. You and Mike,
Bridget, me, the Service Manager, Mel Darwin … Some
time next week, in all probability. I'm not officially back in
the office till Monday, but I've left it with Bridget to
confirm the details. In the meantime she will obviously
accompany Abby on her hospital visits for the moment –
she'll get in touch with you about that. Oh, and I'm going
to be ringing her right now so why don't I pass on the
information about the sister while I'm at it? They can do
what they like with it then, can't they? But *you* forget it.
Casey, *honestly*, I'm sure this will come to absolutely
nothing, so please try not to fret about it, okay? It's just a
process we have to go through. Just think of it like that.
Just a tedious process we have to go through. A box-ticking
exercise we have to be seen to be doing. That's *all* it is. See
it in that way. Okay?'

After I put the phone down I walked back into the
kitchen in a daze. The air was scented with vanilla and it
swirled into my nostrils. Warm cake: one of the best smells

in the world. And then, breathing it in, in deep, measured lungfuls, I suddenly realised I'd forgotten to tell John to enjoy what was left of his second honeymoon, and felt terrible about it. I burst into tears.

Chapter 17

'It's going to be next Monday,' I tearfully explained to Mike over the phone. 'They're all coming: John, Bridget, the Service Manager – God knows who else.' I could hardly speak for sobbing. 'God, Mike – this is going to be all on our record. What have I *done*?'

I'd called him pretty much as soon as I'd finished speaking to John, hoping he'd make me feel better. And he tried his best.

'Love,' he said, 'you just did what you thought was right. That's all. And as far as I'm concerned, there's no crime in that. Okay, so you rushed in a bit, and maybe you should have kept your mouth zipped, but you've done nothing wrong, just remember that, okay? And stop trying to second guess things and jump ahead of yourself. Trust what John said. It'll be fine. What are they going to do to you? Clap you in irons? You've done *nothing wrong*.'

I usually hated it when he pointed out the obvious five times, but in this case he did make me feel better. Whatever the consequences, I'd just have to deal with them when we got to them. I had to stop thinking about it, is what I had to do. It was pointless doing *anything* but try to put it out of my mind.

'God, though,' I railed, mopping my tears with a piece of kitchen roll. 'You know what this makes me think? It makes me think – to hell with bloody fostering! Let them get on with it! I quit! Perhaps I'm getting burnt out. No, there's no "perhaps" about it. How *dare* she complain about me! God, I'm so cross! Do I need all this bloody hassle in my life?'

It was a rhetorical question and Mike knew better than to answer it. He knew as well as I did that I just needed to let off steam. So he just chuntered out a couple more platitudes, promising we'd talk properly about it later; it was pointless trying to get a proper conversation out of him when he was at work, in any case – he was a stickler for company policy and even my 'crisis of faith' wasn't sufficient to make him bend the rules.

I rattled the phone back into its dock and felt some spirit returning. Enough of wailing about injustice. I was just plain old angry now. *Great!* I thought, as I stomped back into the kitchen. This was all I needed. I had a party to help organise, a stressed-out foster child to look after and, on that note, not only did I have to break the news to Abby that she couldn't go off with Kieron this afternoon, I also had to tell her it would now be Bridget taking her to hospital, and do it all without letting my special patented 'mask of calm serenity' slip from my face, while inside I mostly felt like screaming.

And I wasn't at all happy about *any* of it. I couldn't tell her the truth – either about why she couldn't go to Donna's or why Bridget would now take her on her visits – so I would obviously have to come across as the bad guy and feed her a load of nonsense about all of it. Well, thanks a bunch, everyone. Thanks a *lot*.

As it turned out, it was something I was going to have to do sooner rather than later, as well. The phone had rung again, about an hour after I'd spoken to Mike, and this time it was Bridget herself. Only this time I did miss it. The sun was out, and I'd decided to take my upset out on the trampoline – since Jackson and Abby's party was to be at our house, I might as well get it scrubbed up a bit, ready. There was, after all, a small chance that it would be fine enough for them to play outside. If Abby could bear to let them, that was.

I hadn't even heard the phone ring. When I went back in all I saw was the answerphone light blinking, and thankfully – since I really didn't want to speak to Bridget right now anyway – she'd left a garbled message to tell me that, if it wasn't too much bother, Sarah was up for seeing Abby after school. *Well, well*, I thought. There's a turnaround. But I didn't think any further. I was just glad that some benevolent celestial hand had stepped in and provided a reason why Abby couldn't go with Kieron.

I called Bridget back – I had no choice, really – but happily she was in one of her meetings. So I left my own message, confirming that that would be fine, and that she could pick Abby up just after four.

Abby wasn't quite as thrilled to be going back to the hospital as I'd expected. 'But I've just been,' she said. 'Why am I going back again so soon?' I blinked at her, surprised.

'But I thought you'd be pleased!'

'I am,' she quickly answered, presumably feeling disloyal now. 'I mean it'll be lovely to see Mummy, but what about my job at the café? Kieron will be expecting me.'

I winced at the word 'job', imagining how she must have described things to Sarah. I reflected that the truism *was* true – children are *enormously* adaptable. And it was actually a very positive development that she felt this way. It meant she'd adapted so well that spending a couple of hours with Kieron was suddenly her number one priority. I even felt guilty when I turned on the emotional tap.

'Kieron will manage *fine*,' I reassured her. 'And think about Mummy. She's so looking forward to seeing you now she's feeling a bit brighter ...'

I let it hang.

'I suppose,' Abby conceded.

'So,' I said, 'better scoot up and change out of your uniform. Bridget's taking you today, by the way, and she'll be here in fifteen minutes.'

If I'd thought I could just slip that in without much trouble, however, I'd have been kidding myself. So I hadn't. 'Bridget?' Abby asked. 'Why's Bridget taking me?'

'Only because I'm so busy,' I lied. 'It was all a bit short notice, and I'd already arranged to go and look after Levi and Jackson for Riley for a bit. She's got to go out and ... erm ... buy presents for both of you and, um, party food and so on ...'

But Abby wouldn't let it go. 'But I don't know Bridget,' she whined plaintively. 'I won't know what to say to her. Can't you take me, Casey? I don't want to go with *her*.'

'Sweetheart, I can't. Everything's organised now. And Bridget's nice. You'll get on fine with her.'

Abby stuck her bottom lip out. 'But I don't like her! I don't want to go with her! It's not fair!'

I bent down and pulled her in for a hug. 'I know, love. I understand. But life isn't always fair, is it? Just one of those things. You'll be there before you know it ...'

And going with Bridget for the foreseeable future, I thought, but didn't say. We'd cross that particular bridge when we came to it.

Bridget didn't hang around when she picked a distinctly disgruntled Abby up. There was nothing useful we could say to one another while Abby was there anyway, and I suspected she was looking forward to having to deal with Sarah about as much as I was looking forward to my 'super-vision meeting'. And no one's mood had improved any when, three hours later, they returned and Abby marched straight off up the stairs.

Bridget stood on the doorstep and sighed.

'I take it it didn't go well, then?' I asked her. She pulled a face that confirmed it, and I opened the door a little wider. There was nothing to be gained in being inhospitable. I felt sure Bridget felt I'd heaped a load of hassle on her shoulders, but even so we were both playing for the same team. 'D'you want to come in for a coffee before heading home?' I asked her.

But she shook her head. 'I need to get back. Long old round trip, isn't it? And, of course, it's the rush hour. And no, it wasn't the most edifying hour of my life. Abby was *not* happy – well, you can see that – and she's not stupid, either. Whatever you told her, she didn't believe you. Marched straight up to Sarah and demanded to know why you weren't allowed to bring her any more. Which was ... awkward ...'

'I can imagine. What did Sarah say?' I asked her, but then checked myself. Was Bridget even allowed to answer that, or was I now officially out of the loop? It was a wonder, I thought, that Sarah hadn't gone the whole hog, come to think of it, and demanded Abby be placed with different carers. In fact, why *hadn't* she done that?

'Not a lot,' Bridget answered. 'Just told her it was nothing for her to concern herself with and that you couldn't always be the one to bring her, but she's a bright girl – and an intuitive one, too. She picked up on the atmosphere. I think she knew full well that she was being fed a line. Anyway,' she finished, 'I'd better get going. I'm not sure when the next visit's going to be scheduled. I'm not free on Sunday ... So I'll, er, call and let you know, if that's okay. Oh, and just so you know, I'll also be taking her to see her GP. I believe someone's trying to get her an appointment as we speak, but you know what it's like ...' She gave a hollow tinkling laugh.

As I watched Bridget drive off, I tried to feel a sense of camaraderie, of kinship. But I couldn't. I tried, but I couldn't. It also occurred to me that the whole taxi to school business was to do with this as well. It seemed so obvious now. Sarah wouldn't have wanted a foster carer taking her, just in case they – i.e. me – got too pally with the other parents at the school gates. And started telling them things she didn't want them to know ...

Grr, I thought. And because of it – whatever 'it' was – I'd been dumped in all this trouble. All I could think about was that blasted upcoming supervision meeting, and those damning words 'official complaint'. I pushed my sleeves up to my elbows and ticked myself off. *Casey*, I told myself, *this is not about you. This is about Abby*. Then I marched up the stairs. Mike was at the football league AGM, so he was out of the way. And what we both needed was a bout of serious cleaning action.

'Right,' I said when I went into Abby's bedroom. She was sitting on her bed, writing something in her scrapbook. Her bunches were still in place, too, I noted. Good. She put her pen back into her pink fluffy pencil case and looked up enquiringly. 'Casserole,' I said, 'will be ready at eight. And it's now seven. Which I think just about gives us time to clear out the cupboard under the stairs. It's complete chaos. Full of old toys and all sorts of rubbish. It was just our "sling it in if it's got no other home" location when we moved in, and it needs the attention of the sort of girls who mean business. If we're going to have a bunch of toddlers here on Friday, it makes sense to sort some toys they can actually play with.' I grinned at her. 'You up for that?'

Abby was already rolling her sleeves up before she'd even got up off her bed.

'Can I be in charge?' she asked, once we'd got downstairs and opened it. 'You know, decide where everything needs to go?'

'Be my guest,' I said.

Abby smiled beatifically. 'Then I'd better go and get my notepad.'

I had probably taken my eye off the ball. That must have been it – I'd got so wrapped up in trying to unravel Sarah's family tree that I'd lost that extra edge where Abby's ongoing problems were concerned. Our cleaning-out bout had done us both good – no doubt about it. And by the time we sat down to eat I think we both felt calmer.

But the following morning, when Riley came over with Jackson for coffee, I was to realise that my eye had been so far off the ball that you could have put a dozen goals past me.

She'd come over – Levi was now back in nursery, the MRSA crisis over – to find out a bit more about the complaint. Kieron had passed the news on, when I'd called him to tell him not to collect Abby, and she was typically furious about it all.

But we'd barely poured our coffees before it was to become evident that there were other, more pressing things that needed dealing with. I'd just made a jug of coffee – like mother, like daughter – and realised the sugar bowl needed filling. I reached into the cupboard for the half-bag I knew was in there, but it wasn't.

'That's funny,' I said, half to myself. 'Where's the sugar gone?' I rummaged further. 'Well, that's strange. I'm almost sure there was some in there.'

Riley came up and peered over my shoulder. 'Look,' she said, pointing. 'What's that?' She pointed. 'That bag there – that says "sugar". Is it an age thing, d'you think? Should have gone to Specsavers!'

I tutted. 'I can see *that*. I mean the open one. The one I only opened yesterday.'

'Maybe you used it up,' said Riley.

'No, I remember putting it back. I definitely put it back …' I reached for the new pack in any case. And that's when it hit me. The cupboards no longer looked like my cupboards. There wasn't a single opened pack in there at all.

'Now that is strange,' I said. 'I wonder if Dad's done this?'

Riley laughed. 'What, messed up your cupboards? When would that have been? Right after he embroidered you a tablecloth? Anyway, done what? What are you on about?'

And then of course it hit me again. It was obvious who must have done it. Abby. 'Take a look,' I said. 'There's nothing open. They've all gone. Flour, rice, pasta, currants … you name it.'

'So you've obviously had a clear-out and forgotten about it. Mum, I'm worried now. That *is* an age thing.'

'Hey, less of the old lady stuff, madam! No, this is Abby.'

'Abby did this? Well, I must say I'm impressed. You've got her cleaning out your cupboards for you? Child labour, is it?'

I turned around. 'Don't joke, love – that's one of the things her mother's accused me of.'

Riley's eyes widened. '*What?* You have to be kidding me! Accusing you of something like that when she's had her own little Miss OCD waiting hand and foot on her for all these years? The cheek of it!'

'Riley, don't say that. She's ill.' I peered back into the cupboard. 'And so's poor Abby.'

But Riley was having none of my extenuating circumstances. 'I don't care if she's ill. The mother, that is. That's no excuse. And it's so rich. While you're looking after her daughter! What's she playing at? And what exactly did she think would happen to her precious daughter if there weren't people like you and Dad around, huh? Talk about biting the hand that feeds you!'

It took me a while to calm Riley down about it all, especially when I explained all the details she hadn't known yet. I could tell how angry she was, too, because when I questioned the idea of continuing with fostering she didn't even try to talk me out of it. Every other time I'd had a wobble she'd been positivity personified. But this time I could see she was really upset for me. 'Look, Mum,' she said. 'Seriously, Kieron and I think it's really great what you do

– you don't need me to tell you that. But, you know, we've only just *been* here.'

'Been here?'

'*You*. Having a lorry load of grief! Remember Spencer? Don't tell me you've already forgotten why you had to move house in the first place? I mean, it's turned out brilliantly, but just remember what led up to it.'

'I know, love. I do …' I remembered it all too well. The terrible shame of our last landlord paying us a visit that day. He had brought round a petition that most of our old neighbours had signed, demanding that something be done about 'the type' of children we had living at our house. They'd been referring to Spencer, of course, who had caused no end of grief around the neighbourhood. House breaking, fire starting and fighting were just a few of his misdemeanours. No, I certainly hadn't forgotten why we'd moved.

'Well, *exactly*,' huffed Riley. 'Why the hell should you be made to feel like this all the time? Everything you do – *everything* – you do because you care about the kids you get, and if they can't see that –'

'John *can* see that, love. He one hundred per cent can.'

'Yeah, but what about the rest of them? Honest, Mum. This is a load of trumped-up nonsense, and I'll bet there's something going on with that woman that you don't even know about. Don't let them give you trouble, okay? You just stand up for yourself. And then when you've done that, if you want to tell them all to stuff it, you do that. Who could blame you? The cheek of it!'

I felt tears prickling in my eyes watching my daughter so animated and upset on my behalf. And I also knew it was because she could see my own resilience weakening, which wasn't like me. *Casey, you need to man up*, I told myself.

'Oh, I'm not at that stage yet,' I told Riley firmly. 'It'll get sorted. I know it will, and I refuse to waste another moment worrying about it. Far more important things to do, frankly. We have a party to plan.'

And so we did. Though the business with all my cupboard contents still niggled at me, I resolved to put it to one side and concentrate on my own family, because that, in the end, was what mattered most. And Riley and I, list-makers *par excellence*, went into party planning overdrive, committing everything – from the invitations to the music, the food, the decorations, the contents of the party bags – onto our usual array of carefully scribbled lists. Within the hour we had it all organised, written on our matching sheets of paper, which were then carefully stowed into our respective handbags. Roll on the weekend, I thought, as I cast my eye over our expanding guest list, and having my house full of friends and family.

However, it was difficult to stop my thoughts straying back to Abby and how, in terms of her OCD behaviour, there seemed to be something of a backward slide. And that was another thing, I huffed to myself. Where was everyone's sense of urgency? They (whoever 'they' were – both social services and Sarah felt like they were on my case right now) seemed much more interested in my perceived transgressions against everyone than in the business of dealing with this little girl's mental state. Which, as Wednesday became Thursday, was giving me real cause for concern.

I'd got up early – having decided to cram my shower in before either Mike or Abby – and tiptoed across the landing to the airing cupboard to get myself a towel. I opened the door and just stood there in amazement. Normally I just took clean towels out of the tumble dryer, folded them into quarters and returned them to the cupboard. But it was as if the fairies had been and visited overnight. The shelf had now been reorganised into four distinct sections. Each section was devoted to towels of similar colours, and the towels were no longer crudely folded into fours. Instead, each had been folded once lengthways and then tightly rolled and stacked, end facing outwards. They reminded me of those liquorice rolls you used to get as children, all wound up like a pin wheel, with a coloured centre. I carefully extracted one, being careful not to disturb any of the others. The work, clearly, of a fairy called Abby.

When she came down to breakfast I decided to be direct. I was still acutely aware of monitoring the bald patch she'd created, and as I put her cereal down in front of her I stroked her head, exposing it. Thankfully, it didn't seem to be getting any worse.

'Well, now,' I said, picking up the milk carton and pouring some over her puffed wheat. 'What a neat job you've made of my airing cupboard, sweetie. Where on earth did you find the time to do all that?'

She looked up at me nervously. 'Am I in trouble?' But when she saw I was still smiling, she gave me a rueful one of her own. 'I couldn't sleep last night. Not at all. So I thought I'd be useful. So I got up and did some more sorting out for you. Is that okay?'

I sat down across the table from her. 'It's fine, love. Of course it is. But, you know, you need your sleep. The middle of the night's not the time to be doing housework, is it? Especially on school nights.'

'I know. I'm sorry,' she mumbled.

'No need to be sorry. It's just that we could have done those jobs together – like with my kitchen cupboards. You did them as well, didn't you? But you know those are really my jobs; in any case, you shouldn't feel you have to do them.'

She put her spoon down. 'I know,' she said. 'It's just that I know you've been so busy. And you've been so sad –' That caught me short. I kept my mouth shut, however. 'And seemed so stressed, and what with the party, and having so much to do, I just thought it would be better if you didn't have to worry about the house on top of all that ...' She picked up her spoon again, but then seemed to think better of it. 'Casey,' she said. 'You know you shouldn't keep open bags in your cupboards, don't you? I was going to tell you. That's why I had to throw so much away. Did you know that little beetles breed in flour once it's been opened? And you could accidentally eat them ... it's just *asking* for trouble.'

She picked up her spoon again, while I concentrated on not letting my jaw drop. This poor child. She was obviously so tuned into the emotional temperature because of years of constantly watching and assessing her mother and worrying, day to day, if she was feeling okay.

I also felt helpless, and, once again, angry, because I knew nothing would even begin to be done about it till this whole business of Sarah's allegations was out of the way.

Wednesday, I decided, couldn't come soon enough.

Chapter 18

Before I woke Abby up on her birthday morning, I decided I would take a few of the balloons I had bought for the party, and decorate the breakfast table for her. I was pleased that two cards had already arrived in the mail. One, which was fat and squashy, had been franked by the hospital, so I assumed it must be from Sarah, and I imagined the other might be from Bridget, which made me give her a mental brownie point. It was usual for social workers to do this, of course, but given their somewhat new and strained relationship I was particularly pleased to see it in this case. I popped both on the kitchen table by her place mat.

Once I'd also fixed the balloons to her chair, I pulled out the presents from the family that I'd hidden under the stairs – now it was 'properly organised' I knew it would be the last place she'd look – and placed them alongside the cards. Finally, as a special treat (and for me as much as Abby) I made pancakes and syrup for breakfast.

'Come on, lazy bones,' I smiled, once I'd gone upstairs to wake her. She rubbed the sleep from her eyes and smiled blearily. 'Happy birthday, sweetie!' I said, planting a kiss on her head. 'Why don't you get dressed after breakfast today – come down in your jim-jams. I've made you your favourites.'

She roused herself at that. 'Pancakes?'

'And syrup. Just the way you like them. Quickly then, before they go cold.'

Following me into the dining room, Abby squealed when she saw the table. I had added a daisy cupcake with a candle in it to blow out, and also scattered the table with glitter shapes. She spent a moment taking it in. Had anything like this ever been done to her? *Of course*, I told myself. Sarah loved her. That was never in question. Still, her astonishment seemed genuine. She threw her arms around me. 'Oh Casey,' she said. 'It looks so great! Thank you, thank you!'

And for all that she didn't 'do' birthdays very much, Abby certainly tore into her presents. I watched her happily. Sarah's card contained a delicate silver charm bracelet – the present she'd been buying when she'd had her fall in town – with two charms already: a little heart and a diamante star. And our family had done her proud as well. Kieron and Lauren had bought her a lovely silver locket on a chain, and Riley and David a jewellery-making kit. My sister, bless her, had got her a child's baking set, complete with a new apron and natty chef's hat. 'Oh look, Casey!' she cried as she put it on. 'My own set. I can wear these when I go to work at the café!'

I felt a stab of irritation. It was so silly, her not being allowed to go there. I would definitely state my case about that, come Monday. But just as quickly as I thought that, I put it out of my mind. I was more interested, anyway, on what she thought about what we'd got her, which – inspired by what Kieron had done with the picture of Bob – was a virtual pet. It was a hand-held game console in which lived a 'real life' puppy, which would march up to the screen and start yapping till you patted it, and, once you'd programmed it, needed all the attention a real pet did – regular feeds, exercise and lots of love. It had seemed mad to me the first time I'd come across such a thing, but my niece had had one and had loved it to bits.

Of course, Abby being Abby, she immediately started making plans about how she was going to take care of him. 'Oh, he's so sweet, Casey. And I'm going to call him Snowball 'cos, look, he's *just* like a fluffy ball of snow. And you'll have to mind him when I'm at school because I won't be allowed, and, oh God – what if he misses me?'

I grinned at her. 'I'm sure he'll be just *fine*, love. You'll be the perfect mummy for him, and while you're not there I'll be his foster mum. Now, let's get stuck into those pancakes, shall we?'

What with having to set the console to 'pet' her virtual puppy at various intervals in her absence, it was a bit of a mad rush getting ready without keeping the taxi waiting, and I had a moment of anxiety about my 'inspired' choice of present. Would she now – on top of everything else – worry about Snowball all day?

But I put that out of my mind too – she was going to be made better, I felt sure of it. And it was all about dealing with worries, not doing away with them. And besides, I had a party to get organised, didn't I? It didn't matter how much you pre-organised, a party took work, and there was a lot that couldn't be done until the day.

First up, of course, was the cleaning. Riley would be over later to give me a hand with the preparations, but before that I needed to get the place clean. Mike, of course, thought I was barmy for doing this. 'You're mad, love,' he'd said before setting off to work. 'We're going to have a houseful of dirty little toddlers, making a right mess everywhere, and you want to clean it up ready for them. Bonkers, that's what you are, love, plain bonkers.'

'Oh go on, you, get off to work,' I'd chided. 'It's a woman thing. I don't expect you – a mere man – to understand.'

'Woman thing? No, just a Casey thing,' he chuckled, swiftly ducking to avoid a flicking with my duster.

And, naturally, I took no notice of him, because it was my party, and I'd clean if I wanted to – it was one of the few things I felt I could control in *my* life right now. So by the time Abby arrived home again we were pretty much good to go, which meant she could lavish all her attention on her puppy. So maybe not such a bad idea, then, I thought, as I watched her fuss with it. Though Riley and I both couldn't help smiling as she called to us over her shoulder. 'Just feeding Snowball – and then I'm ready to give you guys a hand!'

'All done, love,' I told her, 'and you've got something to do anyway – get out of your uniform and get changed for the party. Go on, off you go. I've laid some clothes out for you on the bed.'

That was her other surprise. I'd bought her another, secret, present: a proper party dress – pink and white polka dot with a net tutu underskirt. I had no way of knowing whether it would be something she'd choose herself, but judging by the *Glee* obsession and the pink obsession generally, I figured that she might, and she did.

'Oh, it's so pretty!' she cried, blushing as she gave us all a twirl in it. Then she ran across and stood on tiptoe to give me a kiss. But the pleasure was to be short-lived, because she was soon looking past me, her intake of breath an indication of what was soon to come.

'Casey, look at *Riley*,' she whispered anxiously. 'She's just given Jackson a *whole* sausage roll!'

I turned and looked at my little grandson happily chomping his way through it. 'It's okay, love. He can eat things like that now. He'll be fine.'

But my words of reassurance were clearly falling on deaf ears. Abby crossed the room anyway, and sat down on the floor with him. 'I'll watch him for you, Riley,' she told my bemused daughter, then promptly took the remainder of the sausage roll out of his hands. She then tore him off a tiny morsel and offered it to him. 'I won't let him choke,' she reassured both of us. Jackson, disgruntled now, tried to snatch the rest back. But Abby was too quick for him. 'Oh no you don't,' she said. 'You must finish what's in your mouth first, and *then* you can have some more.'

* * *

And so it went on. There wasn't an aspect of this party business that wasn't fraught with danger. The balloons were deemed dangerous if they were attached to the backs of chairs, because the older ones could pop them and then the little ones might choke on them. The cakes needed to be passed for an absence of E numbers; any E numbers present and we were courting a disaster, because the kids would 'all go hyper, and we definitely don't want that'. The living-room rug was a potential trip hazard, the kitchen floor a potential ice rink, and every corner of every piece of furniture was 'an accident waiting to happen'. So, by the time the first guests arrived Riley and I felt certain that Abby was already far too stressed to enjoy a moment.

And our prediction was correct. It was like she was the old woman in the shoe. Because there were so many children she didn't know what to do. Her eyes swivelled constantly, alert to the smallest cry or unexpected noise, and no morsel of food touched a lip without her eyeing it concernedly, as if the world would end if she didn't maintain her vigil. If it weren't for Levi, who kept repeating that she was only a 'little mummy', and taking the wind out of her sails, it would have felt like a mini-dictatorship.

In the end it was Kieron who called a halt to the stress of it and gave all the other kids a break. 'Hey, Abby,' he said. 'Could you do me a favour? Poor Bob's been stuck out in the back garden all this time, so I thought, as I've got to nip out and get some more milk, that you could pop his lead on and come to the shop with me.'

Abby, we could all see, was torn by this request. On the one hand, it was a chance to do something with Kieron, but on the other – could she bring herself to leave?

Her responsibilities won out. 'Oh Kieron, I don't think I can yet.' She glanced around her. 'Can't you go by yourself?'

Kieron shook his head. 'No can do, Abs. I need you to watch Bob outside, while I go in.'

'Love, we'll be fine,' I reassured her. Which seemed to swing it. She just needed permission to let herself off the hook.

We took the opportunity to play pass the parcel while they were gone, Riley quickly sorting the music so we could get it done before they returned. She laughed. 'God knows what unseen dangers she might have found,' she observed. 'What with play dough and chocolates and other deadly stuff.' She passed me the parcel. 'And I hope you haven't mentioned the MRSA!'

I grinned. 'You think I'm mad?' We got the game under way.

But for all our levity there was obviously a serious side to all this. Abby's problems were serious. We both knew that. And as the children started handing the enormous newspaper-wrapped parcel from hand to hand, I was about to discover things were even more serious than we thought.

I caught Lauren's eye. She was waving my mobile from the far side of the breakfast bar and mouthing that there was someone on the phone for me. I thought it might be my mother – she and Dad hadn't arrived yet so perhaps they'd been held up. But then I realised she'd have called the house phone. Perhaps Kieron, then, thinking of something else we might have forgotten. But when I grabbed the phone and answered, it was John Fulshaw's voice I heard.

Back from holiday, then. 'John,' I said, wondering if this was going to be about the meeting. 'It's party time here, sorry,' I said, taking myself off into the garden, so I could hear above the music. 'There,' I said. 'That's better. Can you hear me okay?'

'Loud and clear,' he said. And I was just about to ask him about his holiday – I'd rather talk about that than my impending 'supervision' frankly – when he cut straight in. 'Bad news, I'm afraid, Casey.'

There could be worse news? I thought, shocked. Had she complained about something else?

'What?' I asked him.

'Sarah. She's taken a turn for the worse. It's serious. Apparently she's had some sort of reaction to one of the drugs they've been giving her. Anaphylaxis.'

I'd heard of that. I'd definitely heard of that, in relation to bee stings.

'Oh dear, John. And?'

'And I don't know much more, to be honest. Only that I was to call you, because there's a chance you'll have to take Abby up to the hospital. They're going to keep me posted. I just wanted to forewarn you.'

I took this in. God – on Abby's birthday, as well. 'Look, John, why don't I just bring her up now to see her? I mean she was going with Bridget tomorrow anyway. I'm sure Sarah would be glad to see her ...'

'No, she won't. Not right now. Sorry, Casey. I've not made myself clear enough. She's in shock. She's gone into anaphylactic shock. She's on a ventilator. On a life-support machine.'

Chapter 19

The rest of the party passed in a bit of a blur, and for the first time ever I was relieved to close the door on my family and my little house guests. By the time Mike arrived home, after having an unusually late shift at work – *yeah, right* – I had already cleaned up all the mess and Abby was having a soak in the bath. I was glad to have her away from me for a bit, to be honest, as I felt sure she'd pick up on my radically altered mood, hard as I was trying not to show it.

I couldn't get the image of Sarah, lying on a ventilator, out of my mind. It took me straight back to Sophia, and the image of *her* mother on a ventilator, which still haunted me.

So I was glad to see Mike, not least to distract me from my morbid thoughts. I filled him in on the latest news and told him that we were to expect a phone call later on.

His response was typically pragmatic. 'Oh, and just how are you meant to take her to the hospital?' he wanted to know. 'I thought you'd been banned.' Which was a fair point. This was a fairly radical change of circumstance, though. Plus hadn't Bridget said she wouldn't be around anyway?

'I don't know, love,' I sighed. 'Maybe it'll be Bridget who takes her. Or maybe they'll find someone else. But, you know, if Sarah's that ill I think I'd bloody *insist* that I took her. Because Abby's going to *need* me – and then some. Poor little mite. Anyway, John didn't say. Just let's hope it doesn't come to that, eh?'

As luck would have it, Abby was already happily tucked up in bed by the time the phone rang again. I prayed it would be better news as Mike handed the receiver over. 'Please tell me she's getting better,' I begged, before John had the chance to speak.

'A little,' he confirmed. I felt my shoulders drop as he said it. I hadn't perhaps realised quite how anxious I'd been; how much I'd unconsciously been braced for the worst. 'Well, they've moved her to a high-dependency unit, anyway, which I'm hoping means she's out of immediate danger. And they say she's comfortable and showing signs of improvement. She's also been asking for Abby, obviously, so Bridget is going to come over first thing in the morning and pick her up, if that's okay with you?'

'Oh course. But what do I tell Abby?'

'Oh, reassure her, obviously, that things are okay. But also prepare her for seeing her – the message I've had passed to me is that, physically, she doesn't look too great.'

I agreed I'd do so, and once again, as I put down the phone, felt a wash of relief that I wasn't going to have to greet Saturday morning with the task of telling Abby something so, so much worse.

She obviously didn't take things well, however. In this case, though, she seemed less traumatised by her mother's condition (which trauma she was perhaps already used to processing) than by the news that, once again, it would be Bridget who'd be taking her. And this time she was really kicking off.

'No, Casey!' she said plaintively. 'I want *you* to come! I need you to come with me. *Please*, Casey!'

Try as I might, I just couldn't deflect her from this, and by the time Bridget arrived she was furious.

'I want Casey to take me to see Mummy, not you!' she railed at her, before she'd even had a chance to step into the hall. 'Why can't Casey take me?'

'Because I have to ...' Bridget began, equally plaintively, to my mind. She was clearly no happier than Abby about this. And no wonder. It was supposed to be her day off.

'But why can't Casey come with us?'

'Come on, Abby,' I tried to soothe her. 'Let Bridget have a chance to have a sit-down first. She's driven all the way over here, just so she can take you to see Mummy, and –'

'But why can't *you* take me? No one's told me why *you* can't. Why can't you?'

I looked towards Bridget, while talking to Abby. 'Time for a quick drink before you set off?' I suggested. 'Abby, Bridget has to take you, and that's all there is to it.' My tone clear, I went to switch on the kettle.

'So, did you have a nice birthday, Abby?' Bridget tried gamely. 'A lovely party?'

But Abby was having none of it. Where I knew she'd given up with me, she had no similar plan to acquiesce with Bridget. Ignoring the question, she placed both her hands on her hips. 'I'm not speaking to you, ever again,' she said, 'unless you tell me right now why Casey can't see my mummy no more!'

Bridget looked helpless. But she then seemed to make a decision. 'I tell you what,' she said. 'You're right. Why don't we *all* go?' She glanced at me. 'I'm sure that'll be fine.'

Abby's whole demeanour changed. 'Oh can we, Casey? Please?'

Which meant, for all that I didn't really want to – the last person I wanted to see right now was Sarah, and I'm sure she felt likewise – I could hardly refuse. But perhaps I wouldn't actually have to go in and see her. Not if she was currently in the HDU. 'I suppose …' I said. 'Should I phone John first?' I asked Bridget.

'I'll square things with John,' Bridget assured me.

I went back to making the coffees, thinking I'd better go up and change out of my trackies, but when I turned around to tell Abby to get her backpack it was to see Bridget looking completely transfixed.

Abby had obviously noticed a mark on one of my cupboards and was now furiously scrubbing it. She had the cleaning spray in one hand, cloth in the other, and was going at it at something of a lick, a look of intense anguish on her face.

'That looks fine,' I told Abby. 'Love, leave it now and go and get your backpack from your bedroom.'

Abby stopped abruptly, as if coming out of a trance, put the cleaning things away neatly and trotted off upstairs as instructed, though not without patting the door frame several times before she went.

'Is that the sort of thing you were telling me about?' Bridget asked.

I nodded. This was our normal. It clearly wasn't Bridget's. 'One manifestation of it, anyway,' I explained. 'There are lots of others. They're all logged. They tend to change fairly frequently. You get one under control and another pops up. It's a bit of a finger in the dyke situation.'

Bridget sipped her coffee. 'Poor little thing,' she said thoughtfully.

Good, I thought. Perhaps now we'd finally see some prioritising.

Still keen to be left out of the equation today, I had hoped that Bridget would insist that I stay in the car. But, once again, Abby wasn't having any of it. She refused to go inside unless I came too, and it became clearer than ever that she and Bridget hadn't yet developed a bond of any kind. So although I was dreading it, I found myself trudging along the corridor of the HDU, looking for the room in which Sarah was recovering.

I was shocked when I saw her. I think we all were. She looked really ill, and seemed to be covered in big, glassy-looking blisters. I'd never seen anything quite like it. And she seemed as emotionally distressed as she was physically compromised – and clearly put out that she had to face me in such circumstances. She couldn't bring herself to look me in the eye, and I was relieved when Bridget suggested that we nip out for a coffee. 'We'll just be outside,' she told Abby. 'Give you some time to spend alone with your mum, okay?'

I led the way to the refreshments area – now some way distant from where Sarah was recovering – and accepted the cup of reliably grey, vending coffee that Bridget bought for me.

'Well, that was awkward,' I said, sighing. I was simply saddened by the whole sorry mess.

'I know,' Bridget agreed. 'And you know, I'm really sorry for dragging you here, too, this morning. I'm sure it's the last thing you need right now.'

I believed her. And she was right. And there was little else to say. The spectre of next week's meeting still loomed large in my mind, but greater still was the spectre of poor Abby's future. The day must surely come soon when it was properly spelled out to her that there would be no more going home, and no being back with Mummy. That she'd be moving permanently to a new home and to a vastly different life. What hope for her OCD then?

I turned and gave Bridget a wry smile. 'I was so hoping that something would come up, I really was. That Sarah would suddenly admit to a huge, loving family or something, and that Abby could go to one of them.'

'Doesn't look like there's going to be a fairy-tale ending here, Casey. The poor kid.'

'So the sister thing came to nothing?'

She shook her head. 'We can't even go there. I have no idea about the whys and wherefores, but that's her affair anyway ...'

She trailed off, Wednesday's supervision meeting clearly looming for her too. Perhaps I'd misjudged her. This was no fun for any of us.

We sat there in silence for what seemed like an age, and then Bridget stood up and smoothed her skirt down. 'I'll go in and get Abby now. Back soon.'

I smiled gratefully and threw away the rest of my disgusting excuse for a drink while I waited for them to come back. I could see sunshine spilling onto the floor, creating big bright shadow rectangles. It was shaping up to be the first properly bright weekend we'd had all spring so far. But for all that I just wanted it to be Tuesday.

Abby's spirits were no better. She burst into tears as soon as she saw me, and threw herself into my arms, sobbing. 'Did you see her, Casey?' she said, as I stroked her hair and tried to soothe her. 'It's this hospital! It is! They don't know what she needs. She needs to come home so I can look after her, or she'll never get better.'

Bridget and I exchanged our sighs over her head.

I tried hard to keep a positive head on my shoulders as we returned to Bridget's car and, once there, opted to sit in the back so I could keep cuddling Abby, who, after the shock of

Sarah's physical condition, seemed to be fixated now on the hospital and how much she needed to get her mother out of there. 'I can fix her,' she kept saying to me. 'If they'll just let her home. I can make her better. I know I can. Honestly, Casey. We just need to go back home and she'll be fine again.'

There were no words I could say to make any of this any better, so I opted not to. I just held her close to me, and let her cry it all out, and prayed that somehow, something good would happen for this kid.

But if I thought the day couldn't get any worse, I was mistaken. When we got back home I settled Abby down on the couch with her puppy game, and by the time I'd done that, and Bridget had said a quick farewell from the doorway, I returned to where Mike was, in the kitchen.

'She's left this,' he said quietly, handing me a letter. There was nothing written on the envelope and the flap was unsealed. I pulled it out. Headed notepaper. All very official looking. The words jumped out of me, one by one, each more damning than the last. Official meeting. Acting against social services policy. Breach of confidentiality. Inappropriate conduct. Then they began to swim before me, blurring together as my eyes misted. I threw the damning letter across the table. Then, like Abby, I just sat down and howled.

Chapter 20

'What's wrong? What's happened?' Abby looked from one of us to the other. 'Casey,' she asked anxiously, 'are you okay?'

I leapt from the chair where I'd been sitting and lunged for the kitchen-roll holder. Mike had been trying to shush me, but I'd obviously been too upset. 'Casey's fine,' he reassured Abby now, scooping her up into his arms to distract her. 'Nothing for you to worry about, love. She's just got this … um … headache, that's all. She gets them sometimes. Don't worry. It's just tiredness, I expect.'

He kissed her forehead and smoothed her hair, while I pulled myself together. 'Is it a migraine?' she wanted to know. She was still eyeing me suspiciously. 'Mummy sometimes gets migraines. And they make her cry, as well.'

I nodded. 'Perhaps. I think I just need to take some aspirin.' I blew my nose and wiped my eyes. 'And once it does its magic, I'm sure I'll be fine.'

This seemed to strike a chord with Abby. She wriggled herself out of Mike's grasp, then marched across to me and took my hand. 'Come on,' she said. 'You need to come into the living room and lie down on the couch, so I can give you one of my magic Abby head massages. Then you'll feel all right again. Honestly. Mummy says I have magic fingers. And she's right. I'll make you better. Come on.' She jiggled her hand in mine.

Despite myself, I couldn't help but smile. I allowed myself to be led into the living room, and obediently lay down on the couch, as instructed, while she covered me up with a throw. And she did indeed seem to have magic fingers. *It's just a letter*, I told myself. *It's not telling you anything you didn't know. It's just the official language. That's all. Just the official language they use.*

I also reminded myself that, really, I had done very little wrong. That there was a reason why Sarah had it in for me. Well, if not 'had it in for me' (it felt wrong to think in those terms, especially with her lying there so poorly), at least to head me off and try to get me off her case. And though I'd perhaps never know what it was, it didn't matter. I had an answer for their allegations and I would defend myself robustly. And by the time Abby had finished deploying her indeed impressive brand of magic, she'd turned out to be right. I did feel much better.

* * *

But for all the positivity Abby's magic fingers managed to transmit to my head, the state was temporary. Wednesday loomed. How could it not? I couldn't spend too much time feeling sorry for myself, though, not with Abby in the house. There was no getting away from it: her compulsions were getting worse, and I cursed myself that everyone had probably been diverted from the thing that was of most concern here – not whether Casey Watson had or hadn't been gossiping with the nursing staff or using slave labour to maximise profits, but how this child's mental health seemed to be deteriorating.

There seemed little point running around looking for a mainstream foster home for Abby while she was clearly reacting so badly to the circumstances she was already in. It would be something I'd certainly bring up at the meeting, which was to be on Wednesday. To that end, I stepped up on logging everything very carefully. And I needed to – in what was probably a reaction to the events of the weekend, Abby was giving me plenty to log.

The tapping, particularly, was getting markedly worse. 'Casey, we have to step in here,' Mike said, after work on the Monday, having just witnessed some while getting changed. 'Confront all this. Isn't that what Dr Shackleton said? She's even doing it outside now. I've been up in the bedroom watching her from out of the window. She's been round every tree, every bush – at one point I thought she was going to do every fence panel. And I don't think she even knows she's doing it –'

'I'm sure she does. I mean, I know it sort of looks like she doesn't, but if you do mention it she seems well aware she has. And you're right ...' I sighed. 'This could be just the tip of the iceberg, too. She might have a whole load more stress around the corner, mightn't she? Because by Wednesday they might have even found her new temporary carers ...'

'Don't be daft, love. They wouldn't do that.'

'They might! You never know, they might have even decided I'm no longer fit to foster anyway.'

'Casey, that's just daft, love. Don't make this bigger than it is.'

'That's so easy for *you* to say ...' I countered bitterly. Then immediately regretted it. And ticked myself off. One stressed-out person was enough for any household. I needed to concentrate my thoughts on Abby.

So I decided I would, and even though I'd argued the point with Mike, I decided I would change my tack, if only slightly. I wouldn't stress her further by confronting her; I'd just do that interrupting thing Dr Shackleton had suggested, stepping up those occasions where I stopped her carrying out her rituals.

At Monday teatime, after school, she was particularly stressy – seeming unable to settle in the living room. I watched her tap first the door frame, then the coffee table, then the side table, then the windowsill, while the television played to itself. I pretended to be oblivious, sitting flicking through a magazine while she did this, but as soon as I saw her heading for the door – I knew she'd next want to pop out and 'use the toilet' – I jumped up and opened the door, positioning myself between it and the frame.

'You first, love,' I said, gesturing that she should walk past me into the hallway. 'I'm only going up to get my slippers. After you.'

Abby looked as if she might cry, and then stepped back into the living room. 'It's okay,' she said, wringing her hands together distractedly. 'I've just realised I don't need to go yet.'

We both knew it wasn't her bladder but her need for hand washing that needed seeing to, but I stood my ground. She kept glancing past me to the frame. I knew that if I went upstairs she'd carry out the process. 'Are you sure?' I asked.

She nodded, and took a second step back. Now I knelt down, to be closer to her level. 'Sweetie,' I said softly. 'Is it the wood? Do you need to touch it first?'

She looked frustrated now, struggling to find an acceptable answer. I could almost see her mind torn about being honest or denying what was happening. 'No,' she said, eventually, clearly trying for the former. 'Not exactly. It's just the number seven. It's just lucky for me, that's all.'

A lucky number, then. 'So you have to tap everything seven times. Is that it?'

I could see her chin wobbling. She nodded miserably, still glancing longingly at the door frame. 'If I don't touch it seven times,' she blurted out, 'something bad will happen to Mummy! So I have to. And if I don't, then she'll stop getting better. That's why she was so ill. Because of the party – because I forgot!'

I held my arms out to her, and she ran into them, crying hard against my shoulder. I tried to get my head around the tapping schedule she had imposed upon herself. Was she her own worst enemy, in that regard? She'd clearly been battling with two sets of anxieties at the party – worrying about the little ones, worrying about needing to do her tapping ... The poor mite. She'd probably been putting two and two together to make disaster ever since.

I rocked her for some time in the doorway, cursing not being able to just march her down to Dr Shackleton. Perhaps I'd do that anyway and, well, sod them all. But right now I had to think carefully about what I should say next. I eventually loosened my grasp and pulled my head back so I could face her. 'Abby, sweetheart,' I started. 'These are just bad thoughts – no more than that. Bad things happen – we all know that – but they're not to do with you. It's not the things that you do, or don't do, that make bad things happen. When Mummy got sick over the weekend – well, that was just because of the medicine she was given. Her body didn't like it, so –'

'That's not true. It's because I didn't do enough sevens! And it's so hard, Casey, specially when I'm at school. I can do them on my desk, but they don't let us go outside enough to do it, so I can't do it on the trees, and ...'

She broke up again, crying. 'Abby,' I said, 'I want you to listen to me. I have an idea, okay? When you need to do your sevens, you need to stop and think, "Right – I'm going to talk to Casey." Try to think that, and then I can tell you again – these are just thoughts in your head. If you don't tap, nothing bad will happen to Mummy –'

She pulled her own head back now, and looked at me seriously. 'Casey, it's not just Mummy. It's everywhere and everyone. There's bad stuff on the news all the time. And guess what time the news comes on. Go on – just guess!'

I sighed, knowing what was coming. 'Seven o'clock,' I conceded. 'But, love, that's just the news we watch, in our house. On other channels it's on at other times, and, besides, that's what the news is there for – to tell us what's going on, which of course includes some bad stuff, but also other stuff ...'

'But it's mostly bad. And it's on at seven here, so that's a sign. You see? So if I don't do my sevens anything could happen. To Mummy, or Riley's babies, or you or Mike ... I'm just bad luck, I know I am!'

She was crying again, freely. There was so much muddled thinking, yet I couldn't begin to rationalise. This was beyond being rationalised, and it scared me. I resolved that I would give them till Wednesday – till the meeting. And if there'd been no progress getting her to a psychologist, I would *definitely* get her down to Dr Shackleton.

'You are not bad luck, sweetie,' I said firmly. 'You've been the opposite. You've been like a lucky charm for us. It's been ages since we've had such a beautiful little girl living with us, and you've made all of us – all of us – very happy. And speaking of all of us –' I stood up now, hugged her tightly, then released her – 'Kieron and Lauren are coming for tea tonight so we've tea to get prepared. You going to help me?'

Abby sniffed. I could see Kieron's name had cheered her. 'Okay,' she said nodding as she wiped her face with her sleeve. 'And do you think he'd like it if I made him my special cauliflower cheese? I saw you had a cauliflower and I thought it then, too. Does he like cauliflower cheese? We could have chicken and chips too. He likes chicken and chips, doesn't he? But cauliflower cheese as well?'

Drama receded, then. Moment of anguish passed. 'Yes,' I said, grinning. 'What an interesting combination!'

Abby hadn't been wrong about the cauliflower cheese. It was delicious, and it went down a storm. And I was pleased to see that by the time tea was over she seemed much happier. There was something about being with Kieron which really worked for her, and I reflected that some psychological assessment was so important, as there were clearly triggers, and also ways of lessening her compulsions, if only someone would sit down and work them out.

And it was going to happen sooner rather than later, it turned out. With my resolution so firm about getting back in touch with Dr Shackleton after Wednesday, when the phone rang and the caller identified herself as being 'the children's mental health specialist' my brain had me thinking that perhaps I'd already rung him by the power of telepathy alone. But no, it seemed she was getting in touch after speaking to Bridget. So some wheels had finally turned, after all.

Her name was Elise, and she wanted to know all about Abby, so, given the timing of her call – around seven in the evening – it was just as well Kieron and Lauren were there to entertain her. And now I had her on the phone I was determined to cover everything, so I went through both everything I'd observed and what I knew about her which, once disgorged, seemed, in fact, to be quite a lot.

I also told her how I'd been managing the situation up to now, while freely admitting that 'manage' was entirely the wrong word. I knew so little about OCD that, really, I was just scrabbling around.

'No, no,' she argued. 'Sounds to me as if what you're doing is just fine. You know, in cases like this it's not unusual for a child's compulsions to escalate; for them to develop new ones, even, on what can be almost an hourly basis. Today it's those sevens, but tomorrow you might find it's something else entirely. The important thing is to keep calmly doing what you're doing; bring the compulsion out into the open, and try to get the child to take on board that actually she's in charge and that she has the power to fight the thoughts she has. If this is stress related, things will settle once the stress in her life lessens.'

'But what if it's long-standing? I'm really not sure we've got to the truth there.'

'Then that's a whole other issue, but please don't worry about it. We'll cross that bridge when we come to it and, if we do, there are good treatments. Drug therapy, CBT – I'm sure your GP has told you. But let's not jump the gun.

I need to properly assess her. Which is one of the reasons I'm calling, to fix that up with you.'

So an appointment was fixed, and though I felt little the wiser I was at least pleased to know something was finally happening about this bizarre and crippling disorder. But as I rejoined the family, a strange thought popped into my head. My parents, who'd always run pubs, had once again moved to a new area, and, as would happen, once again, I felt isolated and alone. I hated always being the new girl and having to try and make new friends, and would brood on it daily while walking to school. And I would also, I remembered, count the cracks in the pavement. Every day, from our newest place to my new school.

I did this without fail, but one day I was crossing the final road when I almost got hit by a car. I dodged it, and it sped on, and I continued on to school, but minutes later I was gripped by a sudden, intense panic. In my terror, as a result of the near-accident with the car, I had forgotten to count the remaining cracks.

Even though I knew it would make me late for school, I simply had to go back. I had to run back to the place where the car had almost hit me, and then retrace my steps, counting as I went. It was a terrible feeling; I remember being churned up with anxiety. So much so that whatever the consequences – and there would obviously be some – I couldn't go into school without doing it.

I was breaking into a slight sweat even now, remembering. But at the same time, I finally got empathy for Abby.

Sympathy was one thing, empathy quite another. I now felt even more determined to help her. And now there was Elise. Who would make all the difference. Touch wood.

Chapter 21

Wednesday morning arrived all too soon, and so did more sunshine. As I opened the bedroom curtains, I tried to tell myself it was a sign. Perhaps the day wouldn't be as horrible as I was expecting – not with this glorious weather.

I woke Mike up and set the shower going for him. He'd offered to take the day off work to support me – had insisted, in fact – but I wouldn't let him. 'No, you go to work, love,' I'd told him. 'It's bad enough that I'm to feel like a naughty child, without you having to witness it.' He'd finally agreed as long as I promised him that I'd phone the minute the lynch mob had left.

Though it was actually ridiculous to think like that. Yes, Mel Darwin would be there, which was a slightly scary prospect – a bit like being hauled up before the head teacher. But other than that it would just be Bridget and John, for heaven's sake. Bridget, who was hardly Attila the bloody Hun, and John, who I counted as a friend.

Even so, I was glad to pack Abby off to school, because I could tell myself these things every minute of every hour, yet it didn't make any of this less scary or humiliating or downright horrible. Once Abby was gone, however, I had the solution right in front of me. With an hour still to kill before the doorbell ushered in my fate, I could at least do something physical to take my mind off it. Which in my case meant cleaning – a bout of heavy-duty cleaning – and which I did till my arms ached from polishing and scrubbing and the cleaning-fluid fumes caught in my throat.

That done, I checked the clock for the umpteenth time that morning, and returned to the kitchen to get things set up for coffee. I was still trying to decide what sort of signals would be sent out if I used my posh sugar bowl and milk jug when I heard the doorbell. Swallowing deeply, I walked into the hall.

And there they all were. Had they travelled together? I imagined so. John Fulshaw, Bridget and Mel Darwin. John looked his usual self, but the other two looked pretty starchy. Just workday suits, of course, but in some indefinable way, more so. Or perhaps I was just seeing them differently because of this strange circumstance. I tried to fix a smile in place as I invited them through to the dining area. 'I'll just pour these drinks,' I began. 'So, well, just make yourselves comfortable. I really don't know how these things go, so I'll just carry on as normal and …'

'Casey,' John interrupted me, '*relax*. This is just a meeting, okay? So stop looking so nervous. We're not a bloody lynch mob!' *God*, I thought. Could the man read my mind?

But it did the trick. I did begin to feel some of the tension leave me. John had always been good at doing that.

'I know,' I admitted, carrying the rattling tray of pots to the table. 'I'm just a bit nervous, that's all. To be perfectly honest' – I glanced at the three of them – 'I've never been disciplined by an employer before.'

I sat down opposite John, glad that he'd be the one in my eye line, with the two women either side of me. 'Don't mind me,' I smiled at Mel. 'I'll be okay once we're under way.'

'Well, let's get straight to it, then,' said John, a little over-brightly. Very much so, given what he followed it up with. 'Casey,' he said, holding up a typed sheet in front of him. 'I'm just going to read out the full official complaint. And then Mel will add what she wants to say, okay? Just to explain, Bridget is here just to observe, really – that is, Bridget, unless you have something to add?' Bridget smiled and shook her head. So nothing new would be forthcoming, at least. No late additions to the long list of my crimes. 'In that case,' concluded John, 'I think we're sorted. Casey, you'll obviously have the opportunity to respond to the allegations afterwards, and that will be it, basically. Bridget will take the notes.'

It was horrible to have to sit and listen to Sarah's complaint. It had initially been made verbally, and then followed up in writing, though I didn't question how or when or by whom. It was just grim, but in essence no different from what I already knew: I had listened to what she had termed 'idle gossip', tried to grill staff at the hospital for further information, and then taken it upon myself to try to investigate the matter without consulting either Abigail's social worker or herself first.

I had compounded the first crime by acting as some sort of gang boss, recruiting a nine-year-old child to go and work in my sister's café, and apparently expecting her to 'work for her keep'. And finally, I had committed a breach of confidentiality by discussing Abby's current situation 'in a public place with a stranger' and had also been irresponsible in not having gone to one of my superiors, and instead 'traumatised her greatly' by bringing it up with her. The local authority had agreed with this and wanted me to understand that it was my duty to report disclosures of this nature to them and *not* to a child's parent. They were of course paraphrasing, taking most of what Sarah had reported and wrapping it in social services speak so that it didn't sound quite so bad.

When John had finished recounting his litany of misdemeanours, he didn't look at me, but straight across at Mel, and in what was a clearly well-rehearsed two-hander (I imagined then she must have done this many times before) she simply added that she had read and understood the allegations. 'Casey,' she said mildly, 'you should have approached the authority first. I'll give my recommendations after you've been given the opportunity to speak.' I wasn't sure if I should answer. Say 'Yes, ma'am' perhaps? I really did feel that much like a naughty school child.

I felt awful, generally. Set out like that, I really *did* sound awful – some nosey busybody who should have known better. How could I deny any of the charges that had been laid out to me? On a strictly factual basis – give or take some degree and some of Sarah's language – everything John had read out was true. No matter what my intentions were – and they really had been *all* about helping Sarah – I absolutely shouldn't have done it. And I knew that, which was why I could have kicked myself so soundly. Not so much for what I'd done but for being such an idiot that I had failed to think about how they might have been construed.

I looked around at the trio of expectant faces. They were all patiently waiting for me to say my piece. I took a deep breath and cleared my throat, suddenly wishing myself away – to be spirited away, anywhere but here.

But I knew what I would say and I had practised it regularly. I cleared my throat once more, for good measure. 'Okay,' I said, pushing my coffee cup away from me, 'I realise how that all looks. But I promise you, I never set out to upset *anybody*. I never intended to go against any protocol or procedures and I certainly never meant to cause Sarah any distress.' I looked directly at Mel. 'I genuinely thought I was helping. I absolutely didn't discuss Abby in public with a stranger. The woman – Mrs Shelley – was the one to approach my sister, after seeing Abby in her café, and recognising her, and naturally being curious. Not to mention concerned about her welfare, as well. My sister didn't tell her anything that she didn't already know and the woman simply expressed her surprise – as you would – that Abby wasn't being looked after by her family.'

I took a breath.

'I have thought about this a lot, and it's my absolute belief that Sarah got angry because she didn't want anyone to know about her sister's existence. And I also believe it's why I'm sitting here right now. Yes, I do accept that I should definitely have taken the information to someone before talking to Sarah about it – it was in the heat of the moment and it just came out, and it shouldn't have. I was wrong, and I admit that – I realised it immediately afterwards. I can only apologise and assure you that it won't happen again.

'I would also like to make it clear that Abby has never been employed as "slave labour" by my family. She helped at a charity event which my son ran – which she loved. Nothing different from what any child of that age might. No different from helping at a school fête. And which under the circumstances – you're all aware of how fragile her emotional state is – I can't believe anyone would think was anything but beneficial. That she helped out a second time was directly related. She enjoyed herself so much, and pressed to go back so enthusiastically, that my sister let her – as a favour to *me*, to help *Abby*. Which is all any of my family has ever tried to do, just as they all have for all the kids I've fostered …'

Upon which, my voice gave up the ghost. In fact, I was almost in tears now. I swallowed hard. I knew I was just over-emotional because I felt both silly and misunderstood and self-pitying. Why should I even have to defend my actions, when all I'd ever wanted was to do the right thing?

My hands were shaking as I reached to pour myself a second cup of coffee, and I scowled at my cheerfully arranged plate of biscuits. I would have choked if I'd tried to eat anything, frankly, and now felt silly for having put them on the table.

Once again, John had seemed to read my mind. He reached across and grabbed one, and started munching as he smiled his encouragement, presumably waiting for me to gather myself before carrying on. I was done, though. I had said everything I needed to say. There'd be no further justifications from me. If they didn't like what they'd heard, well, tough luck.

Mel, who had been listening and taking notes, cleared her own throat. 'Right then,' she said. 'Thanks for that, Casey. It's really clear that you thought you were acting in Abby's interests. I'm also confident that you also understand that you went against official policy in not informing us before approaching Sarah. As to the other allegations, there is no case to answer,' she said firmly. 'So, in my opinion, we can leave it there. My recommendation is that no further action is to be taken and there is no need to offer you any extra training at this time. The incident, unfortunately, does remain on your record, but your response and your explanation will go in alongside it. Is that all clear, Casey?'

Crystal clear, I thought, hearing that. *Crystal* clear! It would remain *on my record*? I was shocked about that, for sure – it wasn't something that had occurred to me. I couldn't believe that this whole mess was going to be on my record – there in perpetuity, for the entire world to see. I was being dramatic, I knew, but even so it rankled. Because we still hadn't even addressed the whole issue of the reasons why such allegations might be made.

I took a mental leap while Mel, too, helped herself to a biscuit. It was okay. It didn't matter. It was pretty much over. And it had been nothing like as bad as my imagination had been preparing me for. 'Yes, that's fine,' I said to Mel. 'Just as long as I get to read everything over before it goes official. I can do that, can't I?'

To which I did catch a raised eyebrow snaking up over her glasses. I was pretty sure what it meant, too – cheeky mare!

'Well, now,' said John, who was obviously planning on missing lunch. 'Biscuit anyone, now that's over and done with?' I noticed something in his expression, too – a touch of relief. Perhaps, like me, he was pleased I'd got off so lightly. And I remembered that, as a foster carer who worked for his agency, this incident potentially impacted on him too.

Mel stood up, though. 'Not me, I'm afraid,' she said, smiling. 'I have a very irate colleague trying to sort out a case for me, back at the office. But it was nice to see you, Casey, and I hope our paths cross again – though, ideally' – she grinned – 'in different circumstances.'

'Phew!' said John, dramatically wiping his brow, after she'd gone. 'That went better than I expected it to, hey Bridget?'

Bridget was still at the table, finishing collating all her notes. 'It was okay, I suppose. Although you know what? I have to admit that I'm with Casey on the whole "Mum hiding something" scenario. In fact, when I visited her yesterday, to ask if there was anything she'd like to add to this meeting, she said that she'd had a bit of a rethink.'

'*What*?' John and I said together. Bridget nodded. 'Well, as you just heard, I knew Mel had dismissed the whole slave-labour complaint anyway – and who wouldn't? Ridiculous allegation – so I didn't need to bring it up, but Sarah had actually mentioned it. Said that perhaps she'd got the wrong end of the stick about all that, and sort of put it out there that perhaps – since Abby was clearly so keen on going there – it might be okay for her to go down from time to time.'

I had to stop myself laughing out loud. 'Unbelievable! So Sarah thinks about it, and decides that some of my "misdemeanours" quite suit her, so changes her mind. Just like that! It's a shame she didn't rethink the whole complaint really, isn't it?' I realised I sounded childish, but it was out now.

'I know it sounds like that,' added John, ever the pragmatist. 'But actually, well – great! It's what you wanted. Abby seems to really get something out of helping out at your sister's place, and she's also got a strong bond forming with Kieron, so I suppose all's well that ends well, eh? Yes?'

'You see, silly,' said Mike, when I called him. 'I told you it'd be nothing.'

'I know,' I retorted. I was still feeling a bit huffy. It still rankled that anything would be placed 'on my record'. 'But can you imagine bloody Sarah? Retracting all that about slave labour at the last minute and even asking if Abby can do it regularly! Talk about making the system work for you.'

'Casey, leave it, love,' Mike counselled. 'It's done with. It's all fine. It could have been so much worse if she'd really wanted to press it. Let's just be grateful it's done with.'

But it wasn't over, was it? The question still remained. Who was this sister anyway, and what was the story? I was both mystified and intrigued. And I wasn't the only one. The phone rang a couple of hours later, just before Abby was due home from school. It was Bridget.

'I have rather interesting news for you,' she told me.

'Go on,' I said, mentally preparing myself.

'Well, it's just that I've had a telephone conversation with Sarah. Seems she feels terrible about recent events, and puts it down to her being in a lot of pain at the time and not being able to think straight. Anyway, she's keen for you to return to bringing Abby – fine by us – and wants the opportunity to apologise to you personally.'

This almost beggared belief. Why couldn't she have done that all *before* my supervision meeting? 'Really?' I said sarcastically.

'Yes, really. Though this isn't out of the blue. I think she partly feels terrible because, in the light of her allegations, we'd told her we'd look for a different temporary carer. Which was what, at the time, she said she wanted, but she now seems to have had a change of heart. I think she's also worried that you'll refuse to keep Abby anyway, and given that she'll be going into permanent foster care at some point, a further chop and change wouldn't be good for Abby.'

I tried to rein in my anger. Sarah wouldn't have been privy to dates and details, would she? Probably didn't even know I'd *had* the meeting. 'So Sarah knows she isn't going home?'

'Oh, yes, now she's been appointed her own social worker, she does.'

'So now she wants to make things right with me, just so that Abby stays put temporarily? God, did she really think I'd refuse to keep Abby, just to get her back? She has a very low opinion of me, I must say!'

'No, no, Casey,' Bridget was quick to correct me. 'I'm sure she is *genuinely* sorry. I'm just saying that it probably took this to make her see that she was hurting you needlessly, I suppose. Anyway, the main thing is that she's desperate to apologise, and wants to know if there's any way you can bring Abby up tomorrow, so she can do that.'

'Of course I will,' I said. 'It would be pretty mean of me not to, wouldn't it?'

'Well, thanks for being so gracious,' Bridget said. 'I'm sure it's appreciated. I don't know if I'd feel so charitable under the circumstances.'

And I was pleased that she said that, because, well, it made me feel better. Though, in fact, how could I really do anything *but* that? I glanced at my reflection in the hall mirror as I disconnected, very aware that this wasn't just about Abby. I was fit and healthy; I was happy; I had a big, loving family. And, crucially, I hadn't just had the grim news sink in that my little girl – who I cherished – would never really be mine again. Just someone who came and visited me, while I languished in a nursing home. I couldn't imagine how I would *ever* get over that.

Chapter 22

I edged the door to Sarah's room open, not knowing what to expect. In the intervening twenty-four hours or so I had imagined all sorts. I felt confident now that she was going to apologise and, even if she didn't, I'd got over myself now anyway. I wouldn't have wanted her life for all the coffee in Colombia, so to do anything but feel sorry for her would be wrong.

But I still felt there was more she had to say to me. You didn't react so violently when being faced with a name from the past unless you had a pretty good reason. So what was it about this sister that made her so anxious to keep her at arm's length? I had been fostering long enough to imagine the scenario – to imagine several possible scenarios in fact. Had she abused Abby in some way when she was younger? Had she indeed got a criminal past? Been an alcoholic, or a drug user? Or did she have some other skeleton in her closet? Was there some connection between Abby's OCD compulsions and this woman? Some dark family history Sarah couldn't bear to reveal? I was anxious about seeing her again, but mostly I was all ears; there would be *something*, I felt sure. And though it might not change the situation, or help in Abby's future, I had a hunch it would be something she needed to get off her chest.

I'd obviously been right. Sarah just had that look about her, somehow. Physically, she looked a little better than she had when I'd last seen her, thankfully, though her skin was still a mess, the blisters far from healing. Bridget had explained to me that Sarah had had a rare adverse reaction to a dye that they'd injected into her in preparation for some kind of scan. So a double dose of bad luck, and my heart had gone out to her. She tried to push herself up in the bed when she saw us and I could still see the effort involved in moving.

'Hi,' she said. 'Come on in, both of you.' She beckoned to Abby, patting the bed. 'Come on. Climb up, poppet, and give Mummy a big hug. You know what? My bones aren't so sore today.'

Abby duly leapt up on the bed, and I saw Sarah grimace under her daughter's bear hug, and realised she must have understood all too well how hard it must have been for Abby, seeing her the way she had the other day.

I watched, feeling a bit awkward and wondering what was expected of me. I knew that Abby wasn't aware of all the things that had been happening, so Sarah obviously couldn't say anything just yet. So I would just have to stand and wait, feeling distinctly out of place.

'Should I go and get some snacks?' I ventured, finally. 'I could get us all some chocolate or drinks or something, couldn't I?'

'Actually,' Sarah announced, and I could see she had something planned, 'I was thinking my clever little girl here could go and do that today. Now you're ten I'll bet you can reach all the buttons on the machines, can't you? And you're already so good with money – would you like to do that, poppet? Show Casey here just how good you are?'

Abby jumped down immediately, as if already pre-programmed, and reached into the bedside cabinet for her mother's purse. She smiled at me while she did so. 'You just rest your legs, Casey. And I'll bring some surprises back. Mummy loves me to surprise her, don't you?'

By this time Sarah had pressed her call button, and a nurse stood in the doorway. 'Is Chelsea out there?' she asked her.

The nurse nodded. 'Coming now.'

At which point I heard a familiar cheerful voice, and a new face appeared. 'Hey, Abby,' Chelsea said. 'How are you today?'

'She's off to the vending machines,' Sarah told her.

'Is that right?' Chelsea said. 'Me as well, as it happens. Maybe you could show me where they are. I keep forgetting how to get to them from here.'

She didn't need to glance at me. I got it. So that was Abby taken care of. And with her gone, Sarah's smile had gone too. It had been replaced by a look of urgent desperation.

'Casey, where do I start?' she began. 'I am so, so sorry for what I've put you through. I don't know what I was thinking, I truly don't.' She reached out a bony hand to grab mine. Closer now, I could see she'd lost a great deal of weight. 'And before you tell me it's okay, it isn't. I'm honestly not like that at all, Casey. I want you to know that.'

I sat down in the visitor's chair. Her hand still gripped mine, and surprisingly tightly for someone so frail. 'But it *is* okay,' I told her. 'Apology accepted.'

'I don't deserve it,' she said. 'But I have to tell you the truth now. It's hit me, Casey – hard. I've been a complete idiot. I know that now. But perhaps when you've heard me out you'll understand a little and forgive me.'

She was becoming distressed. I remembered this was a woman who'd just been told her only child was going into care permanently, in all probability. And it was humbling. I think I'd have been distressed too. 'Sarah, look,' I said again, putting my other hand over hers. 'I'm *fine* with it now, *honestly*. I know you were just doing what you thought best for Abby – same as I was – and, as it turns out, perhaps we both acted in haste. You've nothing to apologise for.' I meant it as well. This poor woman – who clearly adored her daughter – of course she did – was her mother! Of course she was protective of her. And who knew if I'd have acted any differently? But there was clearly more to it than that, and she needed to get on and tell me. Abby and Chelsea would presumably be back before too long. 'So, what do you want to tell me?' I prompted.

She took a breath. 'I've been an idiot. It just took all this to make me see it. I can't believe I've been so stupid – or so selfish.' Her eyes began to swim with tears again, and I pulled a tissue from the box and gave it to her. She dabbed at the tears angrily. 'But, you know, that was never my intention. I just thought that if I kept everything between us, it would be okay. That they wouldn't take her away from me. That was my only motivation. Can you understand that? I just didn't want anyone taking her away.'

I nodded. 'And your sister?'

'Isn't a bad person. She really isn't.' She seemed anxious that I know that. 'Whatever you might think … *God!*' She laughed a hollow laugh. 'Isn't hindsight a wonderful thing?'

I agreed that it was. 'And?' I prompted gently.

'And I need to make things right, because I'm going to lose Abby now anyway. They've pretty much told me so, and I believe them. Look at the state of me – God, this is such an *evil* disease. Which is why I need to get hold of Vicky. I can't do it myself. I need someone to explain for me …'

'Sarah,' I nudged again. 'What *happened*?'

So Sarah told me. It seemed she'd been living a lie for almost all of Abby's life. And it also seemed that everything Mrs Shelley had said had been true. Vicky, the older sister, was last known to be living about 200 miles away, in London, but there was no guarantee, because Sarah hadn't spoken to her for eight years. That would have made Abby just a toddler, which would explain why she had no memories of her auntie, who, as Mrs Shelley had said, used to be a big part of their lives.

Sarah had got married young, to a man who was apparently a bit of a womaniser; and, taking on something of a maternal role since the death of their own mother, when Sarah was still in her teens, Vicky, six years older had been set against it. Even so, Sarah – blinded by love (and, perhaps, the need to create a new family) – had gone ahead anyway, and married him.

Though she'd always made her feelings clear, Vicky had come to the wedding, and over a period of years had supported her little sister, particularly when the marriage had started going downhill. She'd said nothing as Sarah's husband started messing her around, and also resisted the urge to say 'I told you so' when he was found to have been having an affair. Sarah had forgiven him – 'I *always* forgave him, Casey' – and the two of them had tried to patch things up again. She was a useless wife, she'd told Vicky, and deserved what she'd got. She was tired all the time and never much interested in sex, so really, she told her sister, what else could she expect? Little did she realise – and neither did her husband *or* her sister – that the MS was already doing its terrible work.

Sarah did, in the end, part with her husband. She gave him another chance – she really wanted to make a go of her marriage – and he'd promised her that he wanted to try again as well. But when Sarah found out, a few months later, that he'd seen the girl again, she realised she was clutching at straws. Still at no point did she consider seeing a doctor about her symptoms. Didn't, that is, till they suddenly seemed to worsen; her fatigue grew more intense, she felt sick and ill, and then, one day, while at work, she fainted.

But she'd be led off the scent by something she hadn't anticipated. The doctor told her she was pregnant.

'I just didn't know what to do then,' Sarah told me, screwing the tissue into a ball in her hands. 'We were finished. He'd moved in with that wretched woman now, so did I tell him or not? My first thought was yes – I thought it might be my key to getting him back. But the more I thought about it the more I realised it was a fool's errand to do that. If he didn't want me, he sure as hell wasn't going to want me once he found out I was pregnant, was he?'

'He didn't want children?'

'Oh, we'd discussed it. But you know how things work. He'd said yes, but not yet. It was always yes, but not yet. And I'm not stupid. Even if he'd been desperate for children, *we* were over. So he clearly didn't want them with me. And I'm not naïve, either. It wasn't the MS that killed our marriage. I used to tell myself it was, but only to try and make myself feel better. But I knew the truth. It died a death all by itself.'

'So you never told him.'

Sarah shook her head. 'He had no idea. And that's how I aim to keep it. He could be anywhere, in any case – the further away the better, as far as I'm concerned. Oh, I went through all the usual scenarios – you have lots of time to think, stuck in a place like this, believe me – but what would

be the point? Yes, he might embrace Abby with open arms
– it's been known – but I suspect not. And that "not" isn't
worth the risk.'

'So what happened with Vicky then? You told her about
it, obviously.'

She nodded now. 'Oh, yes, of *course*. Because, of course,
once I'd made my mind up, I didn't *want* to have a baby. I
was struggling enough by then, and it seemed crazy to even
think about having a baby. Oh, no – I was clear.' I could see
her eyes glazing with tears again. 'I wanted an abortion.
And that, I suppose, was where it all started.'

She took a sip from the glass of water on the bedside
table before continuing. It was still bare, bar a picture that
Abby had done for her, and carefully sellotaped to the door
on the front. 'So by now,' Sarah said, 'Vicky's marriage was
over as well.' She smiled a wan smile. 'Two out of two,' she
said. 'Not terribly impressive, was it?' But in Vicky's case
the reasons were very different. She and her husband had
undergone three gruelling and unsuccessful rounds of IVF,
and by the time Sarah had come to her, increasingly sick,
and now pregnant, Vicky was in the middle of divorcing
him, the relationship having buckled under the accompanying strain.

Naturally, Vicky was aghast at the prospect of her sister
having an abortion. How could Sarah wantonly throw a life
away when she had tried so much to create one? It didn't
matter that this wasn't her baby, or that Sarah was single
and unsupported. It would be her niece, and she could
support both of them – she'd absolutely guaranteed that.

So, if reluctantly at first, Sarah conceded to her older sister's wishes. Though she had many reservations (not least her increasingly fragile health – which she by now had attributed to her pregnancy) she at least felt secure in knowing that she'd have her sister there for her.

And, of course, Vicky was. In fact, even before the birth it felt like she had completely taken over, accompanying Sarah to her scans and all her antenatal appointments, and once the baby was born – and Vicky was, of course, present at that too – what had previously felt like support was beginning to feel like a takeover. The sisters lived close to one another by this time, so it made sense for Sarah to let Vicky stay over, so she frequently would; selflessly stepping in all the time, so that Sarah could get enough rest. 'Which I badly needed, believe me. I had no idea what was wrong with me. I just couldn't get out of bed some days. But I just assumed my bone-weariness and lassitude were a normal part of being a new mother.'

What Sarah did know was that she was now in an appalling situation. She hated relying on her sister, but it was becoming increasingly apparent that she had no choice. Eventually, when Abby was a few months old, and Sarah very weak, it was decided that they should think about renting a house and moving in together, and also, at long last, that Sarah actively seek help. She'd developed a frightening new symptom – she was having episodes of blurred vision – and it was this that set in motion a chain of investigations and the damning news that she was suffering from MS.

'It changed *everything*,' Sarah said. 'Everything. Suddenly all the symptoms fell into place. I could almost look back and pinpoint every little thing about it – the times I could barely walk across a room, let alone flick a duster. The times the idea of sex was abhorrent, the business of just being so, so, so *tired* ...' She smiled ruefully at me. 'Having a reason for it all was almost a relief in a way. There was a *why* – it wasn't just me being pathetic. And though the doctors made it clear that, to date, there was no cure, there was certainly treatment – and now I could get some.

'But for Vicky, of course, it changed everything as well. By now – and, God, Casey, I can't blame her now – I *mustn't* – she was faced with a radically different situation. She was seeing an older, divorced guy by then – might still be, for all I know. Might even have married him – and by now she was also caring pretty much full time for both of us, and I suppose she felt – God, I don't know. How can I know what she felt? I didn't ask her – that she was more of a mum to Abby now than *I* was. And I can see why she felt that – she was so desperate to be a mother, and by now it was to her that Abs would run if she needed something. Trust me, that was hard to watch. So it must have seemed obvious to her: now she *was* like a mum, wasn't she? Well, that's the way it seems to me, anyway. And I'd let her do it. I'd just let her take over. Having relied on her so utterly, I could hardly argue with her, could I?'

Sarah glanced towards the door and then back to me. 'But, of course, my diagnosis changed things: it meant I could rethink everything. And I did. I began to realise that, with treatment, I could step up to the plate. You're a mother yourself, Casey, so you know, don't you?' I nodded. 'And I began to feel panicked. I told Vicky there was no way we were moving in together. That I was Abby's mum, and that I was going to take responsibility for her again ... that I loved her, that she'd still be our lives ... I didn't want to shut her out or anything ... but, of course, she didn't see it like that ...'

'So you argued ...'

'Oh, yes. We argued all right.'

'So that was that? You fell out? You never spoke again?'

She shook her head. 'Oh, no – we spoke again. *Lots*. That was just the beginning of it, really. We had a bit of a stand-off, but of course Vicky couldn't stay away. She continued to support me, and I grudgingly accepted that, but by now it was clear that this guy she'd been seeing was not going to give her a baby of her own, and, you know what? I think she went a little mad then. You know, looking back, it all seems so obvious. But back then I couldn't see it with such clarity. All I knew was that she began to put pressure on me. Subtle at first – Abby was walking now, and she'd be saying, "You know, what if you let go of her and she runs into the road? You know, with your eye problem ..." She'd never really spell it out, exactly. It would always be "What if you have a fall?" or "What if you have a relapse and you drop a pan of boiling water?" – stuff like that. Pointing out all the worst-case scenarios. Putting the bloody fear of God into me, basically.'

'To try and take Abby from you?'

Sarah shook her head. 'No, I don't think so, looking back. I did *then* – I thought that was *exactly* what she was scheming. I thought she had this grand plan to steal her from me. But, no, I think she just wanted to take control of *both* of us. She couldn't have adored Abby more, Casey, she couldn't. But when she started bandying the words "social services" around, that's when I saw my *own* worst-case scenario, believe me. It wasn't much of a leap to understand what she'd been trying to drum into me – that, before long, if I continued to try and live alone with Abby, social services would have her taken into care.'

'So that was when you parted company.'

Sarah nodded. 'Pretty much. It all became so obvious then. She wanted to take my daughter from me, so she was spelling it out to me, wasn't she? I was having more regular relapses by then and I realised she was trying to convince me that if I *didn't* let her have her – I was fixated on this by now – then social services would eventually take her from me anyway. Hobson's choice.'

Sarah was crying again now, so I reached for another tissue. This time she took it but just balled it in her fist.

'So I hid,' she said. 'I looked for a new place to rent – by now I couldn't work, and was living on benefits, with help from Vicky – so I found a new place, a little flat, far enough away that I thought she wouldn't find me. I didn't even register with a new doctor.' She looked at me with dark-rimmed eyes. 'What was I *thinking*?'

I placed a hand on her arm. 'You just weren't thinking straight.'

She sniffed loudly. 'And I didn't think straight again for *years*. And now it's happened anyway. Here you are, here I am. And Abby *is* in care, just like Vicky always said she would be ... God, Sarah! Stop it!' She glanced up at the clock.

She leaned forward, then. 'Casey, in the drawer there. My diary. Can you get it out? I've written the last details I had for Vicky on a piece of paper in there for you. I've got no access to a computer right now, but I'm sure you could track her down pretty easily. Even if she's moved I'm sure you could do that. It's not a common surname. And she worked for years at the place I've put on there – see? That practice of physiotherapists ...'

'She's a physio?'

Sarah nodded. 'I know. Ironic, isn't it?'

'But what about your cousins? They'd know where to track her down, wouldn't they?'

'Oh, I doubt it. We were never a close family. We barely knew them. And after Mum died ...' She looked down at her hands in her lap. 'Well, let's just say I'd be surprised if they even remembered our names. So, no. I don't think so.' She looked imploringly at me as I pulled out the piece of paper. 'So, do you think you could? Could just *try*? I'd be so grateful. I can't even bring myself to dial that phone number. I really can't. But if you could just try ... tell her what I've told you. Tell her I'm sorry. Tell her ...'

I looked at the paper now. 'Oh, this is a London address. Were you in London?'

Sarah shook her head. 'No, that's where she went. That was the last time I was in touch with her. She'd tracked me down, of course. She wasn't going to give up that easily. But I didn't want to know. I refused to see her, refused to speak to her, to answer her letters, and the last thing was that she wrote to me, telling me she'd been offered this post in London, and that she'd happily turn it down – and I'm sure she meant it – if I'd only let her back into our lives. I told her to shove it.' Sarah sighed. 'Like you say, I wasn't thinking straight. Don't think I've been thinking straight ever since. Except finally, *now* …'

'Don't worry,' I said. 'I think I know what to tell her. I'll do my very best. Though, Sarah, you know, I have to tell someone about this. Protocols …'

She smiled a wan smile. 'Stuff protocols, Casey. I mean, do whatever you have to. But if you can find my sister I'll never be able to thank you enough. I've sacrificed too much of Abby's childhood already, I have to make this right again. I *have* to.'

I don't know if Chelsea had been waiting just outside the door with Abby, but it seemed that just the right amount of time passed – time to mop tears, time to regain composure – before the two of them were back again. We'd been talking for almost an hour by now, and Sarah looked exhausted.

'Are you okay, Mummy?' Abby asked anxiously. 'Did they change your leg dressings okay? Do you want me to check –'

Sarah shook her head. 'They're all fine, poppet, honestly.'

I glanced at Chelsea, who mimed holding a phone to her ear. 'Anyway,' she said brightly, 'I'm afraid I led Abby somewhat astray while you were tied up. Do we confess, then?' She looked at Abby, who giggled.

'We had chips!'

'At this time?' Sarah chided. 'You'll have spoilt your tea now, young lady.'

'Oh, I dare say we could have it a little later,' I said.

'And what about our surprises?' Sarah said. 'Did you remember the surprises?'

Abby's hand flew to her mouth. 'Oh! No, we didn't get you anything!'

'I'm not hungry,' Sarah assured her. 'But you know, I'd love a new book. How about you get me one of them instead?'

Abby didn't need asking twice.

'Thanks, Chelsea,' Sarah said, as soon as the door had closed behind her. 'I really appreciate it.'

Chelsea smiled warmly. 'Any time,' she said.

'And, Casey, obviously don't say anything to Abby – not just yet. Not until I know there's any point.'

I felt a surge of energy. I would do my darndest – after observing all due protocols, obviously – but I would do my darnedest to make sure that there *was* a point. To my mind, there couldn't not be. I thought of Donna, I thought of sisters. Like puppies, you had them for life. There *had* to be a point.

Ten minutes later we were back in the car, pulling out of the car park, my mind in overdrive, brain whirring with everything Sarah had told me. All of which I had to keep under my hat right now. All of which could make the biggest difference imaginable. I smiled to myself. Drug user, criminal, abuser ... instead, what we had here was just an issue of territory. That and a surfeit of love. And a surfeit of love was almost always a good thing.

I glanced through the rear-view mirror to see Abby's eyes meet mine. She grinned. 'It's so great that you and Mummy are friends again,' she said.

I laughed. 'We were always friends, love.'

Abby waggled a finger. She really did have such a lot of emotional intelligence. 'Oh no you weren't,' she said knowingly.

I laughed again. 'You are one funny onion, little Abigail. Now what say we play some really loud music, all the way home?'

'Yay!' she said brightly. 'And we'll sing along too. But you mustn't dance.'

'Mustn't I?' I jiggled in my seat. 'Not even a little, like this?'

'Not at all,' she said. 'Old ladies look funny when they dance.'

So that was me told. We headed home.

Chapter 23

Too late to do anything about the sheet of paper I now had safely tucked into my handbag. I would have to wait until the morning before I could sort anything out. But I was fit to burst, so by the time Abby was in bed and I could at last fill Mike in properly about Sarah's revelations, it tumbled out of me like the Niagara Falls.

'You are not going to believe what I have to tell you,' I began, practically dragging him into the living room, and turning down the volume on the TV remote at the same time.

'Oi!' he protested. 'I wanted to watch that.'

'You can watch it on Plus 1,' I said, throwing the remote onto the sofa. 'Oh, Mike, you are not going to believe this.'

'Well,' he said. 'Tell me then. What exactly is it that I'm not going to be able to believe?'

I poured out the whole story, hardly pausing for breath. 'See?' I said. 'I knew she was hiding something about that sister of hers. I knew it!'

'And you were right,' he conceded. 'Well done, Dr Watson. But let's not run away with ourselves. You haven't found her yet, have you? And even if you do, there's still no guarantee she'll want to know.'

'Rubbish,' I said. 'Of *course* she will. How could she not? She's her sister. She *loves* her.'

Mike grabbed my hand and squeezed it. I looked down at it. 'What's that for?'

'For being you,' he said. 'Just for being you, love.'

Mike was right, though. He always was. Nothing was guaranteed here. And it wasn't just a case of Vicky being amenable to helping out, either. Social services would see it as a positive – I felt sure of that – but in terms of Abby's future it was more complex than them saying, 'Cheers, then! Over to you!' Abby was now officially in the care of social services, and now they'd taken on that responsibility they had a duty of care. You didn't simply hand children back to people, just because they happened to be relatives. The usual protocols would obviously need to be followed. To be less than thorough – to check that Vicky would be a positive influence in Abby's life; to assess her properly – would mean they were failing in that duty.

'But my hunch is they'll jump at it,' I told Mike. 'Isn't yours?'

'And you think she'll be up for just moving in and taking over and them all living happily ever after, just like that?' Mike countered. 'Would it *really* be that likely? I imagine she'll have her own life to think about. She could be married, have kids …'

I flapped a hand to silence him. 'Shh,' I said. 'Positive mental attitude, okay?'

No, it probably couldn't help. But neither could it hurt.

I was too excited to sleep properly that night. And the next morning – the hour that I spent with Abby before school – seemed to stretch interminably. I was trying to be as normal as possible, but was operating mostly on autopilot. And Abby being Abby, she could tell something was up. 'Casey, what's wrong with you this morning?' she wanted to know. 'You're all fingers and thumbs today, like Mummy.' She narrowed her brows. 'You're not having trouble with your joints, are you?'

I laughed out loud at this, but she was clearly still concerned I was making light of something serious. 'You're not doing things right, Casey. Look – you've put a knife next to my cereal bowl instead of a spoon, and you've put the milk back where the orange juice goes. Do you know that MS can come on all of a sudden?' She frowned at my bemused expression. 'Casey, it's not a laughing matter.'

She really didn't miss a trick, and it was bittersweet to know it. 'Silly me,' I said. 'It's because I stayed up too late last night. Me and Mike watched a scary movie and then I couldn't sleep.'

This seemed to convince her. 'Ah,' she said. '*That's* why. I have nightmares if I watch something scary. You could always press the "i" button on the remote – that tells you all about the programme that's coming on. That way, you'd know if it was going to be something scary, and then you can choose something else.' She tutted, and I imagined Sarah saying all these things to her. All these little life skills she had needed, which I'd never even thought about. She really had turned into such a singular child. Oh, I thought, but wouldn't it just be so wonderful if she could return to being an ordinary one now?

Abby opened the fridge and restored the contents of the door to their rightful positions. 'There,' she said. 'The way you are this morning, you'd have probably poured orange into your coffee.'

I called John first, and then redialled and got in touch with Bridget. Happily, today, she had no meetings. She was as pleased as John had been to hear the news – not to say surprised. And she couldn't see any reason why I shouldn't try to get in touch with Vicky, since that was what Sarah had asked me to do.

'And maybe, assuming you do get hold of her, you could give her my number. If she wants to be brought up to speed with what's happening, I can also then put her in touch with Sarah's social worker, Andrew. I'll call him in the meantime and fill him in.'

'I will,' I promised. 'So – any suggestions on what to say?'

Bridget laughed. 'Not a clue! I mean, how *do* you start a conversation like that? But knowing you, Casey, I'm sure you'll come up with something. I can't imagine you ever being lost for words. Good luck anyway, and give me a ring back to let me know what she says.'

This meant that nothing now stood between me and that piece of paper, which contained three phone numbers – one I knew was about fifty miles away, one down in London and one mobile – plus the name of a private physiotherapy clinic. All I had to do now was pick up the phone. But now I felt strangely nervous.

Mad, I thought, making a very naughty decision. Mike had recently brought a swing seat, in preparation for our first summer in our lovely new garden, and since the sun was out I decided I would sit outside and have a cigarette, and make the calls from there. I'd not had one in ages, and I had no intention of falling off the wagon, but right now it would steady me to make the call.

I ferreted around above the freezer, found my stash, grabbed my coffee and, with the phone tucked under my arm, went outside.

I'd only smoked half the cigarette before deciding I didn't really need it. What I needed, I realised, was to just get on and do it. So, placing my coffee on the grass beneath me, I dialled one of the numbers, opting, for reasons of positive mental attitude, for the local home phone. The one I most feared would be the wrong one.

'Okay, what did you forget?' a cheerful female voice answered.

Which completely took me aback. 'Oh!' I spluttered. 'Is this Vicky?'

Now the woman had to change gear. 'Oh, I'm sorry,' she said, flustered. 'I thought you were someone else! Yes, this is Vicky. Who is *this*?'

A. Maz. Ing. I thought. *Bingo.* First strike and I'd got her. Well, someone called Vicky, anyway, and what were the chances? 'My name's Casey,' I told her. 'Casey Watson. You won't have heard of me …'

And then I began to tell her about Sarah.

To this day I can't remember exactly what I said, but I do remember that, despite all my careful rehearsals, I ended up blurting everything out in one seemingly endless stream. This produced a result that was so spectacularly pleasing that I couldn't help but do a secret high five to myself. She was crying, then apologising for crying, then laughing, then thanking me and making me go over everything again.

'I can't tell you how long I've waited for this day to come,' she told me. Then she laughed. 'Actually I can,' she said. 'About seven and a half bloody years! How is she? How is Abby – oh, I can't believe she's ten now! Does she still look like Sarah?'

'Yes, she definitely looks like Sarah. She's just a sweetheart …' No point in going into detail at this stage. One thing, one bombshell at a time.

'You didn't go to London, then? Sarah was so sure you'd go to London.'

'Yes, I did, for a trial, but I hated it down there. And I kept coming back to Abby. Suppose Sarah changed her mind? I'd given up trying to track her down by then, but I knew she had my number, and that maybe one day, if she needed me, she'd get in touch. I'd not burned my boats anyway – just rented my house for three months. So back I came. Oh, I can't believe this. I really can't!'

'Sarah thought you might have married the man you'd been seeing ...'

Vicky snorted. 'Fat chance. Let's just say I had my fingers burned in that regard. No, I've been in a relationship, but it didn't work out. It wasn't really going anywhere. I'm assuming you know about the whole IVF thing ...'

'Some,' I said. 'I'm sorry ...'

'But let's not dwell on that. What do I need to *do*? In the here and now? Which hospital is she in? Oh, God, I know it sounds crazy, but it's so good to hear she's okay. I mean, I know she's *not* okay, but I'm sure you can imagine what I've been thinking ...'

Yes, I told her, I could imagine all too well.

Of course, there were still plenty of hoops to be jumped through. Pleased as I was with Vicky's reaction to my phone call, it was important I still said nothing to Abby. Much as Vicky obviously wanted to do what she could for her niece and sister, you couldn't expect someone to just drop her whole life and embark on a new one. And it seemed to me, judging from what little I knew of Sarah's long-term prospects, that in order for Abby to avoid being placed permanently in the care system, that would be pretty much what she'd be required to do.

In the short term, however, my priority was to tell Sarah. I'd explained to Vicky that Abby was currently being fostered by me – and what my role was – and that social services, now her legal guardians, were looking for a permanent placement for her, since the home situation was no longer tenable. I gave her Bridget's number, and also told her about Andrew, Sarah's social worker, and that if she spoke to both of them she'd have more facts than I had, particularly as regarded the MS. I also told her that, as far as I knew, Abby didn't even know of her existence; that if she knew anything it would only be that there had been someone called Vicky in her life once – which was the only thing, I think, that really upset her.

'Oh, my,' she'd said, after an audible exhale of breath. For a moment I wondered if it would be a deal-breaker. I tried to imagine being in her shoes, given the amount of care she'd lavished on her beloved baby niece, and how it must feel to know the child in question didn't even know of you, let alone love you. But she rallied. 'I suppose that was the only way,' she added. 'Under the circumstances.'

'I think you're right. Under the circumstances *then*,' I agreed.

But when I tried to get hold of Sarah on her mobile, I failed. I tried half a dozen times, left messages on voice-mail, and eventually decided that she was probably having some treatment, and that I'd wait for her to pick up my messages and get back to me.

Which she duly did, mid-afternoon. 'Oh, Casey, I don't know how to thank you!' she told me.

'Thank me?' I said. 'I haven't even told you my big, big news yet!'

Sarah laughed. 'You don't need to. I already know it.'

'How come?'

'Because Vicky's already called me!'

'She has?'

'Called me right after she spoke to you. That very instant.'

Which was the best news I could have wished for. There was still a string of hurdles ahead, obviously, but the finish was in sight. We had definitely jumped the first of them now.

And we were half way over the second one as well, it transpired, because Vicky had apparently also spoken to Bridget and Andrew, and was keen to hear what she could do.

'One step at a time, of course,' Sarah said, 'but they certainly seem amenable to having a meeting to discuss what would need to be done to ensure Abby wouldn't need to go into care. I mean, I know she *is* in care – and I can't begin to thank you enough, Casey – but if we could halt this horrible process, find a way to get back home again …'

'It would be the very best news imaginable,' I agreed.

'But don't say anything to Abby yet, will you?'

'Oh course not. Your call, I think.'

'Because I've asked Andy – Andrew, my social worker – if he'll go to my house and pick up some pictures. I thought I should sit Abby down and explain things to her, show her all the photos, tell her what happened. I need to be honest with her. If we're going to make this work, I have to be honest. She needs to know why her auntie has been out of her life for so long.'

I felt for Sarah. It wouldn't be a pleasant job for her because, ultimately, she had to take responsibility for it having happened. But children are adaptable. Programmed to love unconditionally. I said so.

'I hope you're right,' Sarah said.

'I don't hope,' I reassured her. 'I know.'

There was also the small matter of where home would be, and how it would happen. Could Sarah even *get* home again? Or was she too sick? No, it was the right thing to keep Abby in the dark for a little longer. Just until some of these concerns had been addressed. No rush. It would be too cruel to offer the child a lifeline, only to snatch it away again at the last minute.

'Frogspawn!' Kieron announced, standing on the doorstep with two empty jam jars, both of which he had accessorised with string handles.

It was Sunday afternoon, the back end of a full-on weekend. With no word from anyone – bar from Bridget, on the Friday, with the usual 'we'll keep you posted' – the Watson family was in something of a state of limbo. Well, I was – the rest seemed blissfully unaware of my inner angst, Abby because she had no idea how radically her life trajectory might be changing, and the rest because they'd all obviously taken one of my son's infamous 'chill pills'. As Mike had observed more than once, what would be would be.

But I'd had to provide Abby with plenty of distractions – this trip to the woods being one such – if only to divert her from worrying about me, and how unusually distracted I seemed. I felt sure she'd reverted to her earlier diagnosis: that I might have MS, and didn't know it.

For all that I'd smiled at her, it really brought it home to me that this child was hard-wired to expect the worst, always, that life was a very bumpy, uncertain road, one on which bad things had already happened and were certain to keep happening, to the end. Things also hadn't been helped by her most recent visit to see Sarah, where Sarah too – like me, in fact – was struggling with the business of having such momentous news, but which she couldn't yet share. She was waiting for Andrew to stop by with the photos he'd promised to get for her. There'd been no real change in the atmosphere – none that I could detect while I was with them, anyway – but Abby was almost superhuman in her sensitivity to the emotional temperature, and half-way home she had burst into tears.

'Mummy's going to die!' she sobbed. 'Isn't she?' And she wouldn't be pacified. In the end I'd had to leave the motorway so I could calm her down properly, she was just so convinced there was something her mother wasn't telling her.

She was fine again now – an evening phone call had calmed and reassured her – and since then the weekend had passed smoothly enough, though her rituals were as evident as they'd ever been. How would the coming developments affect her, I wondered, as I watched her. For the better or, actually and quite possibly, for the worse? I tried to put it out of my mind, and keep her occupied – she'd been to the pictures with Riley and the little ones, been out shopping for clothes with Lauren, been to Donna's café for lunch (and had the promise of another 'shift' there next week) and now here was Kieron on the doorstep, as we'd planned, making good with the aborted frogspawn outing, which was actually sensible, as it had turned out. If they'd gone before it would probably have been too early.

'You up for it then, Abs?' he said. 'For getting those hands of yours dirty?'

Abby blushed scarlet, to the roots of her hair. She really did have a full-on Kieron-crush, bless her.

And, getting ready, I was pleased to see she was actually quite sanguine. 'It's better to go now,' she said, reaching into the under-stairs cupboard for her wellies. Since she'd been with us, there was no messy pile of outdoor footwear in there. Wellies were corralled into a row, in tidy pairs, each clipped together by a clothes peg. 'Casey, I'm surprised *you* didn't know about doing this,' she'd exclaimed.

'How come?' I asked now. 'Because some might be turning into tadpoles?'

Abby shook her head. 'No, because it's *dry* now. So we won't get all yucky. That's *why*.'

They returned an hour later, largely free of mud, as promised, the jam jars duly half filled with the clear wobbling gunk.

'And we don't need to wash it, do we, Mum?' Kieron ask me.

'No, of course not,' I said, confused. 'Why would you wash it?'

'See, Abby?' Kieron said. 'I told you. She doesn't believe me, Mum. She thinks you have to wash the jelly off.'

'Of course you don't,' I told her. 'They need the jelly. That's what they eat.'

Abby looked mortified. 'Euww!' she said. 'How revolting! They actually *eat* it?'

'They actually eat it,' Kieron said. 'You eat jelly, don't you?'

'Yes, but not jelly from a pond, stupid.' She punched his arm playfully. 'Strawberry jelly, raspberry jelly –'

'No,' Kieron said, ever the pedant, ever quick with details. 'Like the jelly you get round the meat in the inside of a pork pie. It's like *that* jelly.'

If possible, Abby was even more disgusted.

'Kieron, that's just *gross*! You're actually making me feel sick now.'

'Abs,' he laughed. 'Man up. You are *such* a lightweight.'

It was another good hour before the frogspawn was sorted, Kieron helping Abby prepare the tank to provide just the right environment, which I was pleased about, since it would be me who had to deal with the lion's share of looking after them, I didn't doubt. It had been ever thus. It was also great that Abby now had something on which to base her school show-and-tell the following week.

And Riley too did a stint of helping out. Once Kieron had left, and I took my gorgeous grandsons up for a bath, she helped Abby draw some pictures of the newly acquired frogspawn, and helped her write a project piece on frogs and reproduction, which she could use for her talk, along with some of the frogspawn, which we'd left ready, for the time being, in its jar.

By the time I came down again, however, they'd moved on to colouring, the two of them carefully filling in a lovely riverside scene, which in this case was destined for her scrapbook. I felt a real glow of love for my children, as I watched them. And a pang of sadness that poor Abby had no siblings. But the moment passed; she's soon have a new person to love her, wouldn't she?

I let the boys go and join them while I went into the kitchen to prepare some tea, smiling to myself as I watched them all gathered around the dining table, and marvelling, as I often had, with all the kids I'd fostered, that this little family tableau looked so, well, so very *normal*.

I said as much to Mike later that night, once we'd gone to bed. 'And it's weird, isn't it?' I added. 'Whenever I get that feeling, that's the very moment I realise.'

'Realise what?'

'That that's it. That's the exact time you know it's all coming to an end.'

Mike thought for a moment. 'Well, that would seem to figure,' he said finally. 'Sign of a job well done, I'd say.'

'Fingers crossed,' I said. 'I'd hate it if she had to stay in care now. Let's just pray that the whole Vicky thing works out.'

And even as the irony of doing it wasn't lost on me, yet again, feeling slightly foolish, I touched wood.

Chapter 24

To say I was on pins all Monday morning is something of an understatement. I'd sent Abby off to school with her jam jar and her nerves about public speaking, and I was actually quite glad she was so preoccupied by it – it meant her focus wasn't entirely on me.

In my mind what was coming would be simple. Sisters reunite, aunt meets niece, everyone loves each other, Abby can live with aunt and they all live happily ever after. You don't often get fairy-tale endings in foster care, but I really couldn't see why not this time.

It was eleven before Bridget was back on the phone, however, by which time I'd done everything domestic I could think of, including checking on the frogspawn and feeding Snowball, the virtual dog.

'So,' she said, 'I gather you know all about the telephone reunion? It's fabulous news, isn't it? Who'd have thought it?'

'Yes, it is,' I said. 'And?'

'And are you free tonight, basically? Sarah wondered if you could bring Abby up to see her after school today, so she can sit down and tell her about her auntie.'

'Of course,' I said. 'More than happy to – I'm bloody useless at keeping secrets. She's got the photos from Andrew, then?'

'Yes, and she's keen to get on now. As is Vicky. She's travelling up here tomorrow.'

'And then?' I asked.

'And then we'll talk about ways we can play this. Too early to second-guess things – we need to explore the options. But for the time being we've put a hold on the search for a permanent foster home – at least till we get some idea of what's viable. Sarah's needs are complex. There's a lot to think through. And as yet we don't know how big a commitment her sister's prepared to make. It's not something you can expect a person to dive straight into. Not without considering all the implications, as you know.'

Even so, I spent the afternoon grinning. I knew I was programmed to look on the bright side – had been like it all my life – but even taking that into account, I really couldn't see how Vicky – from what Sarah had said of their history, and from how she'd been with me – would want to do anything short of whatever was needed.

I still had the grin on my face when Abby got home from school. So much so that, half-way through telling me about her frog-reproduction presentation, she stopped speaking and stared. 'Casey,' she asked, 'have you bought me a present?'

I was puzzled by the odd question. 'A present? No, sweetheart, I haven't, I'm afraid. Why would you ask that?'

'I don't know yet,' she said, after a moment's consideration. 'You just have a very funny look on your face. The one Mummy used to have if she'd got me a surprise.'

I grinned. 'Well, I suppose I have, actually. In a way. We're off to see your mum tonight –'

'I thought we were going tomorrow?'

'We were. But now we're going to go tonight instead. So that is a surprise, isn't it?'

She still looked suspicious. 'Hmm, you're still hiding something, Casey. I can tell.'

I shook my head. 'I really don't know where you get your ideas from, Missy. Now come on, let's get that frogspawn back into the fish tank, then off upstairs to get changed, so we can have a snack and still beat the rush hour.'

Abby was still suspicious when we arrived at the hospital and called the lift. 'Casey,' she said, wriggling her hand away from my own, 'your hand is all sweaty.' She scrutinised me carefully. 'Are you sure you're not coming down with something?' If she'd been tall enough I don't doubt she'd have checked my temperature as well, by placing a hand on my brow.

'No,' I said. 'I'm not. I am honestly not, I promise.' And I made a mental note, such as I'd made many times before. A life of crime and subterfuge was definitely not for me.

Happily, however, the wait would soon be over, but not before Abby had one last moment of panic, seeing her mother's equally strange expression as we approached her. She looked from one to another, than popped her hands on her hips, as she often did. 'Mummy, Casey's being all weird. Why's she being weird? Do you know? Look –' She pointed. 'Look at her face.'

Sarah smiled. She looked better today, her skin returning to normal. And also better in a way that was impossible to define, but was there nevertheless. I waved hello.

'Well, poppet,' she said to Abby, 'I think we can allow Casey her funny look today. I have one too.' She gently turned Abby's face to look at her. 'See? And that's because I have some very special news for you.'

My cue, I decided. 'I'll pop off then,' I said. 'Grab a coffee …'

'No, no,' Sarah said. 'Please. I'd really prefer it if you stayed.'

'Oh, I think this is between you two,' I said, feeling very much that this was private – between the two of them. But Sarah insisted. 'I want you to be part of it – that's if you don't mind – just in case Abby has any questions later on. You know, if she forgets anything. It's going to be a lot to take in.'

And, of course, she was right; that *did* make perfect sense. So I sat down on the visitor's chair – Abby climbed up onto the bed – and listened quietly for the next half an hour while Sarah told Abby the whole story. It was punctuated once or twice by questions from Abby, but mainly she listened intently while her mother talked, taking everything in – I could see her processing all the details – in what appeared to be a very matter-of-fact way.

I found the way Sarah spoke a little odd to begin with. She seemed to speak to Abby more like she was a friend, rather than her daughter: she was straight to the point, and wasted no time on dressing things up. There was no kiddie-speak, there were no euphemisms, just the bald, unvarnished facts, which I felt might be a little strong for a child of such an age.

But then I thought some more, and it occurred to me that this was probably how it had always been. This was probably the dynamic Abby was used to. And it was a hunch that was confirmed when Sarah finally finished speaking, and Abby, having digested it, announced her verdict. Again it was matter of fact, unemotional, pragmatic. 'Mummy, you've been so silly. All this time, and I had an auntie I didn't know about! If you'd made friends with her, I could have had a break once in a while.' She patted her mum's hand. 'But don't you worry,' she continued. 'Now you're friends again, it's all going to be okay, isn't it?'

Wow, I thought. She really was such a singular little girl.

Of course, both of them then started crying. And, feeling a bit teary myself now, I decided to leave them to it. Outside the room I took a deep breath and fanned my face with my hand, then set off down the corridor towards the vending machine. As I fiddled around in the bottom of my bag for some change, Chelsea joined me. She had her coat on, presumably done for the day.

'Great news, isn't it?' she said, smiling at me. 'About the sister turning up.'

'The best,' I agreed, pressing the button for the disgusting gunk that passed for coffee. 'Well, in theory. There's still no guarantee they'll get either of them home.'

'Oh, it'll be fine,' Chelsea said. 'Trust me. We're already on the case. Having a family member on hand makes a *world* of difference. We're already looking into setting up the whole external package. You'd be amazed at the stuff you can get these days. You have to remember, keeping a patient in their own homes, rather than in *a* home, is the outcome that works out best for everyone. Not an option while there's no one to support the patient, obviously, but now that's not the case –'

'You sound pretty confident that's going to happen.'

Chelsea shook her head. 'Not just confident. I've already been in touch with Vicky, haven't I?' She patted my shoulder reassuringly. 'So not just blind faith. But I expect you probably know all the gen anyway.'

I couldn't help but smile at that. Albeit ruefully.

Chapter 25

After promising to return the next day, and holding a clutch of family photos, Abby was eventually persuaded to leave the hospital. We'd be back the next day anyway, so she could finally meet her auntie. Just call me Parker, I mused, as I helped her strap herself into the car.

She was still full of excitement when we finally made it home. We'd hit the tail end of the rush hour, and to compound things it would also soon be Easter, and though Abby hadn't broken up yet, the motorway was choked with caravans and heavily laden cars. So Mike was already home by the time we arrived back, and, as I'd predicted, she couldn't wait to pounce on him with her news. I'd never seen her so excited, I thought, but then, why would I? She'd come to us with the weight of the world on her shoulders. Now it was being lifted, and, lighter of heart, you could see the sunny child she could become.

'And, you know what, Mike,' she babbled on, having shown him all her pictures, 'Auntie Vicky might even move in with us! And then everything will be just perfect – she'll be just like Mary Poppins. She'll do all the cleaning and the cooking – well, once I've shown her how to do it, anyway. And then I won't have to do a thing, hardly. Not a thing! Won't I, Casey?'

I laughed at her analogy, even though privately I was thinking *whoah there!*, starter guns and jumping them springing immediately to mind. But now was not the time to quash her hopes. Who knew, anyway? From what Chelsea had said that was a distinct possibility. Instead I stroked her hair, mindful that that bald patch still existed. 'You're just like a mini Mary Poppins yourself, love. Practically perfect in every way.' I scooped her up for a hug then. I did need to say *something*. 'Hey, but you know, Abs, let's not even try to imagine how things might be *just* yet. We need to speak to your aunt first, don't we? Make sure that she's able to help.'

But Abby was having none of it. She wanted this too badly. This meant everything. This would mean that she and her mum could go home. 'Oh don't worry about that, Casey,' she told me, throwing her arms around me. 'Mummy said Aunt Vicky will love me. And that's because I can charm the birds!'

'Well, it's certainly looking positive, by the sound of it,' Mike said, once Abby had skipped off, at his suggestion, to get her paints and her sketch book, and perhaps make a picture to give to her aunt the next day.

I filled him in on what Chelsea had said, which to my mind made all the difference. 'And if they're already at that stage, I think we're right to feel positive.'

'Well, I'm still keeping everything crossed – and so should you. You know how these things can change at the last minute.'

We both did – and well. In that case, though, the change had been the best we could hope for; our last foster child, Spencer, was headed right up to the last minute for the last place I wanted him to go: a residential unit, a place where they send out-of-control teenagers. And he'd been younger than Abby, even – just nine years old. Going home had been out of the question for poor Spencer. Or so we'd thought. Within a fortnight things had taken a dramatic turn, and he'd ended up living happily with his mum.

He still was, and, God willing, would continue to do so. So was it too much to ask that things turn out well for Abby too? I hoped not, and, actually, though I understood Mike's caution, I thought it would, at least in the sense that her aunt would now be there for her. Nothing I'd seen or heard made me anxious about that.

But that was only half the picture. Not even half the picture really. Sarah still had MS – a particularly nasty type, too, and would presumably continue to deteriorate. And Abby herself, for all our temporary euphoria, still had a complex set of psychological issues, none of which – no matter how much we might pretend otherwise – could be instantly magicked away.

Abby's very excitement gave me cause for concern. It seemed all so black and white, and why wouldn't it? She was a child – she didn't deal in grey areas, in much the same way as she hadn't a few days earlier. If Sarah came home, then, as night followed day, she'd get better. This was the thing Abby had hung on to since she'd been with us. And why wouldn't she think that anyway – over the years her mum had been ill many times, and each time there would be a corresponding well period. So she could process what she'd seen in hospital by applying the same logic. She was ill, but soon she wouldn't be. And then all would be well.

It was this more than anything that concerned me: that, actually, Vicky didn't quite know what she was taking on in Abby. Sarah herself didn't seem to have the first clue, come to that – and that posed another problem: that, in the haste to reconcile the family, the severity of Abby's condition might get sidelined, which might make her worse, which might throw everything else into disarray. And this could also – I'd done enough reading for me to know this might be true – make her OCD more entrenched, and possibly permanent. It was such an insidious and tenacious thing to have.

I couldn't sleep that night. Mad, given how tired I was – but it was like I was in overdrive now. This was a situation that would very soon be out of my hands, but if there was one thing I could do it was to focus on Abby, and do the best I could – assuming Vicky wanted my input about her niece – to give her as much helpful information as I could.

Mike was snoring, too, which was pretty much the decider to get up. I struggled to get back to sleep at the best of times when Mike was snoring, and with my head so full of thoughts it would be impossible tonight. So, instead, I went downstairs, poured myself a glass of water and turned on the laptop, determined to do anything I could to make it easier for them.

I spent a good couple of hours sitting bleary eyed at the kitchen table, making notes, jotting down web addresses, stacking up the printer queue with things to print out in the morning, as well as collating my notes, updating them and jotting down anything I thought might be useful. And while I was reading a web page, specifically aimed at children with OCD, I came across an article that seemed particularly useful – it was all about support groups for young carers. Clicking onto a link, I was thrilled to find that there were such groups sprinkled all over the country – and that they held regular meetings that young carers could attend, both to share their experiences and also to meet new friends just like them; friends who, unlike all the 'childish' ones Abby knew, understood and empathised with each other's problems.

It was an eye opener for me too – the numbers were really something. It seemed that thousands of these young kids spent most of their lives looking after a parent, which left them little time or inclination for socialising. After a little more research, I was even more excited to find that there was actually such a group only about a mile from where Sarah and Abby lived. I couldn't quite believe that they had lived the way they had for so long, when a support network had been practically on their doorstep. If only Sarah had done things differently. It just all felt so sad.

The following morning, if not exactly refreshed, I felt rested. And with a to-do list that Abby herself would have been proud of, I also felt ready both to gather the fruits of last night's furious labour, and catch up generally with my mounting piles of paperwork. If this placement was to end soon – which was beginning to look likely – I needed to be sure all my notes were in order and that anything new I had of Abby's, such as her forthcoming appointment with the psychologist, needed to be put into her file. All that done, I phoned both Bridget and John, to update them, and to confirm that we'd meet Sarah at the hospital around five – Vicky, *en route* now, would already be there. And of course to ask if either had heard anything else. But they had nothing new to report other than that Vicky had set off and she would be at the hospital with Sarah from about 1 p.m. that afternoon. According to Bridget, she was very much looking forward to meeting me later.

But, of course, I'd forgotten about Kieron.

'Hello, love,' I said when he suddenly appeared in the kitchen, having bellowed out his usual hello. Though I was always pleased to see him, I hadn't been expecting him, and as it was out of character for Kieron to do *anything* without planning it I was confused to see him now. I said so.

'Am I losing the plot?' I asked as I automatically reached for the kettle. 'Or is there something I should have remembered about today?'

Kieron pulled his hoodie off and carefully slipped it over a chair back, before pulling it out and sitting down on it himself. He glanced up at the clock. 'No, no,' he said. 'I just thought I'd come early. I've had nothing on today at the youth club, and Lauren's in college, so I thought I'd wander down, that was all.' He eyed the open laptop. 'You're not busy, are you?' He looked at me anxiously.

'As if!' I laughed. 'Never too busy for my lovely boy, you know that!' Which was not only the required response, but also true. Early, though? Early for what? I was confused now. There was clearly something he was early for. What had I forgotten?

And then the penny dropped. Shit! I'd forgotten about the café shift. With everything else that had been going on I'd completely forgotten that I'd arranged – and with both Donna and Kieron, hence his arrival – that Abby would spend a couple of hours helping out down there tonight.

'Oh, love,' I said, grabbing mugs from the cupboard, 'I'm such an idiot. We've got to go to the hospital when Abby gets home – to see Sarah. It's only just come up, all this, and it's all been such a big deal that I'd completely forgotten about you picking Abby up.'

I explained what had happened in the last forty-eight hours, and how it looked like Abby's Cinderella story was to have a happy ending, with Auntie Vicky playing the role of Fairy Godmother. And as I explained things I watched Kieron's face begin to change. By the end he was looking positively gloomy.

I sat down and brandished coffees and placed a hand over his arm. 'Hey, why the long face?' I asked, 'as the barman said to the shire horse ...' This at least raised a hint of a smile in him.

He shrugged. 'It's just sad,' he said simply. 'I'm going to miss her.'

'Oh, love,' I said. 'But you knew she'd be leaving.'

'I know, and I spoke to Riley and she did say about this auntie ...' He sat and pondered. Then shrugged again. 'I just feel sad.'

Looking at Kieron, you wouldn't know. Well, you might, but you probably wouldn't. You wouldn't fully appreciate, not unless you knew him like I did, that for all that he looked so normal – so tall, blond and, yes, ridiculously handsome – he was actually different, in myriad ways, from most of us. Even I forgot that sometimes, like in the last few Abby-centred weeks. I'd been so touched by how positive an effect knowing him had had on her that I had neglected to consider what their friendship meant to *him*.

As with lots of things about Asperger's, it had slipped under the radar. Of course he'd be sad. He found it difficult to make friends, too – how could I forget that? And though he had a great group of close friends, and a wonderful, caring girlfriend, making a connection with another human being, however unlikely, in terms of age, and then losing it again – *God, Casey*, I thought, *of course he's bloody sad!*

'I know,' I said, 'and I can see that, and I know how much you're going to miss her. I'm sure she'll miss you as well.'

He sipped his drink. 'It's hard,' he said having clearly thought. 'All this fostering. It really was kind of like …' he trailed off, and I could see he was trying to articulate something.

'Kind of what?' I coaxed.

'Kind of like having my own little sister. We really got on, Mum. And, bloody hell, it was sooooo good –' now he grinned at me – 'having a sister not bossing *me* around, for a change!'

I laughed. 'Hey, don't be too down. I have a suspicion about Abby. Now she's got a big brother in her life and a part-time job at Truly Scrumptious, I suspect we'll still be seeing plenty of her, don't you?'

And I wasn't just saying that either. I believed it. It could be arranged – assuming all parties concerned wanted it to, at any rate. No, we didn't know what would happen to the family long term, but, as of right now, Sarah didn't live so very far away.

'Anyway,' I finished, 'Abby's going to be here soon. So perhaps before you leave for work you can let her know when your next shift is. I'm guessing she'll be keen to do one. She's not even had a chance to get her birthday chef's kit out yet. And, love, remember what I always say –'

'What? Not "Rome wasn't built in a day," Mum. You *always* say that.'

'No,' I tutted, 'good proverb though that is. No, I was thinking more that "endings aren't always necessarily endings". So put that in your pipe and smoke it.' I paused. 'Though, obviously – here's another for you – don't smoke.'

It didn't make a blind bit of difference, obviously, but an hour and a half later, at the hospital, seeing the three of them together for the first time, and seeing how alike they all were, kind of did.

Fairer than her younger sister, Vicky was even more like Abby than her own mother was, and I could tell straight away what a strong bond aunt and niece would have – from the aunt's point of view it was already a given.

And Vicky had an air of older-sister authority which, though it might have contributed to the break-up between her and Sarah, straight away convinced me would now serve them all well.

'Abby!' she greeted her niece, leaping up as we entered. 'Oh, sweetheart, I am so glad to see you again!' But she didn't overdo it. She seemed to have a sixth sense that, for all Abby's excitement, facing this virtual stranger in the flesh would be a very different matter. So, instead of over-whelming her with hugs and kisses, she let Abby take the lead. Which she did, formally extending her right hand towards her aunt's. Vicky shook it with a warm smile but equal formality.

'Very pleased to meet you too,' Abby said shyly.

Vicky turned to me then. 'And you must be Casey,' she said, extending her own hand to shake mine now while Abby went to hug her mother. 'I owe you such a debt of thanks, I really do. And I can't tell you how pleased I am that you had the guts to stand up to my sister.'

'I think I'm going to second that,' Sarah added. At which both of them laughed. And I did too. What did a flipping 'record' matter anyway? It was just words, stuffed away in a drawer, after all. This was a real-life happy ending, and *I'd* made it happen. Surely that was what mattered. Given a fair wind and a glass of wine with Mike later, I might even spare a few minutes to feel pretty damned proud of myself. It didn't matter that it might have happened anyway, eventually; equally it might not have, so grabbing at least a slice of the credit felt only fair.

Not that there weren't still a few hurdles to jump over. Though it seemed everything was moving in the right direction, Vicky still had a life of her own to live. But she seemed to have already spent time thinking that through. Her house, she explained, was already on the market. 'Downsizing. Coincidence or destiny?' She laughed. 'I'll take either. Seriously, I was at a crossroads –' She turned to Sarah. 'I'll tell you later. And, one way or another,' she said, turning back to me now, 'I was going to make a change. So this has kind of crystallised my thinking, which is actually a big weight off my mind. I can stop bloody procrastinating now!'

Then I saw her glance at Abby, and didn't really need to know any more. Her eyes shone with tears and her expression spoke volumes. There could be no better incentive for her, clearly.

Chapter 26

As often happens when you foster – my kind of fostering, at any rate – decisions get made, and it feels like it's all go, and then there's this period of inertia. Which is right. Because where a child or children's lives are concerned, no decision should ever be made in haste. So, confident as everyone was that this new plan would be workable (for Vicky, initially, to accompany Sarah home from hospital, once the necessary support arrangements were put in place), it was important that all the boxes were ticked.

Most of this was outside my remit. These were things that would be handled by the medical team, including Chelsea. She, along with Vicky, another physio, seemed to really know her way around the system, as did Andrew, Sarah's social worker.

Vicky would also, meanwhile, be assessed by social services, so that when the time came – and this all rested on Sarah settling home again without difficulty – she would already be formally approved as Abby's carer. This wouldn't be a full check, such as was done on all potential foster carers, like Mike and me, but something less formal – what was known as a friends and family assessment, and which was less intrusive and only took a couple of weeks – less, perhaps, given the circumstances and everyone's will to push things on.

The will was certainly there, and not least of all on my part. Abby duly attended her appointment with the child mental-health psychologist, and it was agreed that once Abby was settled more permanently somewhere she'd be referred to someone close by for a fuller assessment, at which point a plan of therapy would be agreed. In the meantime it was agreed that it would be useful for Vicky if she spent some time with me so I could discuss Abby's needs in more depth.

We arranged it for the following Thursday. Abby, who'd now seen her aunt three times at the hospital, couldn't wait to see her again. 'Oh, I need to do her another painting,' she gushed as I filled her in on Wednesday night that Vicky would already be at ours when she got home from school the next day. I'd arranged for Vicky to come to us mid-afternoon, so we could talk through the rituals and compulsions and so on, and how best she could manage them herself. She'd have professional input, of course, and very soon I'd be bowing out, but forewarned was forearmed and we were of a like mind regarding that.

'That would be nice,' I said.

'So I'll start it now, while I'm in bed, and then I'll get up extra early so I can finish it off before school. But I'll need glitter. Will I be able to get out your box and use your glitter? It'll need to be extra early, and I wouldn't want to wake you and Mike up. I know you need lots of sleep once you're older.'

I laughed. 'Tell you what, I'll go down and get it out right now. That way it'll be all ready for you in the morning.'

She smiled. 'I'm going to make it a special "going home" picture. Ooh, I'm so excited. Do you think it will be long now?'

I didn't know, so I couldn't tell her. 'Not too long,' I reassured her anyway. Inwardly, even as I said it, I felt strange. Strange, yet at the same time the feeling was familiar. Much as I wanted a child to leave me in such happy circumstances, and get finally settled somewhere permanent, there was always a part of me – a selfish part – that wished they'd be slightly *less* happy at the prospect of saying goodbye and moving on.

We covered this in training, of course – children in care often had huge attachment issues, and, with a history of abuse or neglect, being able to move on was a key defence mechanism. If they allowed themselves to attach too easily, they were often storing up more heartache – being able to detach easily was not only a result of years of being unloved, it was also sometimes the only thing that kept them sane.

This wasn't the case with Abby. She was going home to be with her mother. Her aunt as well – why on earth wouldn't she want it to happen sooner rather than later? But it didn't make it any easier. It was just plain old hard, this job, I thought. You did all you could to reassure the kids that they would be going home – and, at the time, you really meant it. But then, when it came to it, no matter how professional you tried to be, a little bit of you wanted them to be upset about leaving you. Not at all what a foster carer should be thinking, of course, but most definitely what the mummy inside of you always felt.

I leaned down and kissed the top of her head, then brushed the hair to one side to check her bald patch. Was it my imagination or did there seem to be a little new growth there? Wishful thinking, perhaps, but I didn't care – I could see it. 'Not too long,' I said again. 'Night, night. Sleep tight. Don't let the bed bugs bite.'

Abby groaned, as she always did. And then she made me laugh out loud. 'Casey, you know me. They wouldn't *dare* to!'

When Thursday afternoon came around, however, I was to get a wonderful reminder that attachments can reveal themselves in other ways.

Vicky and I spent a productive hour running through things together, and the more I talked to her the more I liked her, and the more I felt confident that here was someone who'd come through on any promise. Nearer my own age than Sarah, and having followed a roll your sleeves up and get on with it career in the health sector, she really couldn't be better placed to head up this little family – the little family she'd always wanted to take care of, however overwhelming her enthusiasm in the early days. Once again – this happened often – I reflected on family life, and that families really did come in all sorts of unlikely configurations – all different, some surprising, but so many of them perfectly functional. And this one – right down to Snowball the virtual puppy and youngest member – looked like it could function as well as any other.

Abby flew in from school just as excited as I'd expected. She even stopped to hug her aunt before flying into the toilet. That would mean nothing to anyone else, but it blew me away. For as long as I could remember now, this had never happened. This was a first. She also came home with plans, which she'd clearly been thinking about all day.

'Casey,' she wanted to know once she'd done her hand washing (which happened afterwards), 'I was wondering, do you think we could take Aunt Vicky to the woods before we have tea? I want to show her the frogspawn.'

'But the frogspawn's here,' I said, confused. 'You can show it to her now.'

'No, not that frogspawn,' she said. 'I want to show her the rest of it. Show her where we got it. I'm sure it'll still be there. And if it's not there'll be tadpoles anyway. Pleeease?'

I couldn't think of a single reason why not. It was a lovely spring afternoon, and we'd been sitting at the table for ages. If Vicky wasn't in a hurry to rush off – which it seemed she wasn't – then why not? It would be good to stretch our legs. Though a thought occurred to me. Did Abby really even need or want me there?

'You know,' I said, 'you don't need me to come with you. You can take Aunt Vicky on your own if you like, while I start on tea. You're such a big girl now. And you know the way.'

Abby shook her head. 'No, I want you to come too,' she said firmly. 'Please, Casey?'

'Well, I guess tea can wait,' I said. 'Go on, then. Get upstairs and get that uniform off. I'll write a note for Mike, so that if he comes in he'll know where we've gone.'

It was lovely going back into 'our little wood' (as I liked to think of it) and see it so transformed by the spring. There were a few bluebells still out, and the pungent scent of wild garlic, and, a far cry from the dripping, gloomy place we'd first brought Abby, it was full of growth, bright and verdant, in the dappled afternoon sun.

You could hear the stream babbling even before you could see it.

'Careful here,' Abby warned, grabbing my hand as we walked down the bank. 'It gets steep here,' she explained to Vicky, 'so you have to be very careful and watch your step.' But it was clearly no longer her own step she was watching. It was mine. 'You'll be okay,' she continued, to Vicky, 'but Casey has to be careful because she'd older.'

'Hey, cheeky!' I protested. 'Less of the older, please, missy. I'll have you know that not so very long ago I used to go rock climbing – real rock climbing, not over these tiddlers. And caving, as well. And,' I huffed, 'lots more besides.'

Abby gave me the sort of look that made it obvious she doubted that *very* much, but then spotted something that made her stop and lift her arm. 'Stop here!' she demanded, and then turned to us dramatically. 'Because we're here. I want to show you a secret,' she added. 'Both of you.'

She let my hand go, then, and leaned down towards the jumble of stones, then reached down and – to my surprise; I wasn't even sure if she had her hand gel – manoeuvred two large, moss-covered rocks out of the way. She then pointed. 'Can you see?' We both peered down to look closer. She'd revealed a third one beneath them – a flat rock which was embedded in the muddy bank. 'That,' she said proudly, 'will be there *for ever*.' She then leaned even closer to inspect it, and gestured that we should. She stepped back, to let us see better. 'Can you see what it says?'

Vicky and I shuffled closer to the edge and duly looked. Etched into the rock, in black marker pen, were some words. I read them aloud. 'Kieron and Abby woz here. BFF.'

I then turned to Vicky. 'As in Kieron, my son.'

Abby quickly replaced the rocks and put a finger to her lips. 'But it's a secret. We're not really supposed to write on rocks. It was just a wild and crazy scheme of bonkersness, Casey.'

I laughed out loud, but she shushed me again, and then added, as an afterthought, 'Oh, and if you don't know what

BFF means,' she said proudly, 'it actually means "best friends forever".'

It was tricky balancing on the rocks by the stream that afternoon, but not half as hard as wrestling with my emotions. There were just too many of them, all at once, and in such a confined space. Thoughts about Abby, this poor isolated, different sort of child. This child who couldn't connect with her peers in any way. This self-professed child who didn't have friends, and now did, and it meant so much to her that she'd brought us here to prove it. Then there was Kieron, who also found it so hard sometimes to understand people, and for whom such an unlikely bond had been formed with this odd little girl. And who would miss her. Who was sad that she'd be gone. And about me, and what I'd said to him only the other day. Yet another mum-mantra, a few words to get him to feel positive instead of gloomy. And which actually – coincidentally – had turned out to be the right ones. This proved it. Endings *aren't* always necessarily endings.

For Abby, Donna's call came completely out of the blue. For us it was anything but.

It was two weekends later – the end of two frenetic weeks. A date had been arranged for Sarah's discharge from hospital. The trial now finished, and with a comprehensive care package now in place, she would be returning home, with Vicky, the following weekend. She would have a full team of therapists allocated to her, as well as a nurse and a physiotherapist, both of whom, initially anyway, would visit her on a daily basis. Both Andy and Chelsea – and everyone else – had moved mountains; Chelsea in particular, Vicky told me, had spent literally hours with her – and Vicky too, so she knew how best to support her.

And that mattered. Sarah was so used to hiding her condition that it was almost a reflex to pretend all was well when it wasn't. And it was important that she accept how things were, rather than how she wished them; as Chelsea had said, that's what would keep her out of hospital.

Abby herself was scheduled to return a week later, to give her mum and aunt time to properly settle back in. The house needed to be cleaned from top to bottom, and specialist equipment installed, such as hoists, a stair lift and a whole range of small adaptations, not to mention a state-of-the-art wheelchair. Most importantly, however, it needed to be stripped of the accoutrements that had been put in place so that Abby could run things. That, to my mind, was the most important thing. It was time for Abby to reclaim her childhood.

And if we needed evidence of that importance, we were about to get it.

'Hmm,' she huffed, shaking her head after speaking to Donna. I'd called her specially to let her know the call was meant for her. 'She wants me to go into work this afternoon. Just like that!' She was actually quite cross. 'Doesn't she realise that I'm busy with my packing to go home?' She put her hands on her hips, and I had to cover my mouth so she couldn't see it. 'Honestly,' she said, 'she's got to get used to not having me around. She can't rely on me all the time – I'll be too busy!'

I kept my hand over my mouth till she was back upstairs, gone to fetch her pinny. Only then did I properly dare breathe out. Mike rolled his eyes. 'And there goes the little madam that we've grown to know and love, eh? Do you think we've created a monster?'

I laughed, though quite quietly, just in case she was listening. 'Just call me Dr Frankenstein ...' I said to Mike.

As indignant as our little master chef was about being 'put upon', her face when we arrived at the café was a picture – marching into the café, pinafore tied neatly around her waist, hair tied too – in her regulation plaits. She stopped dead in her tracks as she tried to take it in, blinking, stunned, as the whole family shouted 'Surprise!'

And not just our family – behind the cakes and balloons and 'Good Luck Abby!' banners, there was her mother, in her wheelchair, hair all done, make-up on, looking lovely. Taking our lead from Sarah, then Abby, then Vicky, then Donna, we all caved in and allowed ourselves to cry.

It was a wonderful afternoon, obviously, but also tinged with sadness. I knew Kieron was working hard to hold it all together, and it was sweet to see the way Abby clung on to her BFF, holding his hand, patting him and asking if he was okay. She was still a little mum – even if it was to a six foot two 'boy'. And it wasn't just Kieron's welfare that she was concerned for, it seemed. That night, as I tucked her in, she pulled my ear close to her lips. 'Casey,' she said, 'you'll be okay when I'm gone, won't you?' And I could barely speak enough to reassure her that, yes, I would.

And then, somehow, it was time for her to actually physically leave us, and when the day dawned – as always happened, so why the hell didn't I get used to it? – I had to steel myself all over again. Which I did, and it was fine, and it was over, but it really wasn't. Because I'd overheard Kieron saying to Abby the very night before, endings weren't always necessarily endings.

'Don't worry, love,' consoled Mike as we trooped back inside, and he did what he always did – popped on the kettle. 'I'm sure John Fulshaw will be back on the phone before you know it. Shall we take bets on how soon? Next week? Tomorrow?'

'I know,' I agreed, dredging up a smile. 'You're probably right.' I mentally shook myself. Time to let go. 'And I'm okay. *Really*.' I reached into the dishwasher for some mugs. 'And who knows what he'll have for us. I wonder if it'll be a boy or a girl next time?'

Mike folded his arms across his chest. 'I don't know, Case, but here's what I'm thinking. It'll either be a boy, or it'll be a girl. I'd say it's fifty-fifty, either way.'

We went to bed that night not realising that the 'next time' we'd joked about was actually right around the corner. And, as it turned out, even with that fifty-fifty chance of getting it right, we could never have guessed what was to come next …

Epilogue

Two years on, Vicky still takes care of Sarah and Abby, who is now twelve, in high school and doing well. Though her mother's illness continues to make her home life challenging, the support they receive from Vicky, the NHS and social services means she is no longer isolated, and can live a full life.

She's got something of a social life now too. And she has also been something of a star: we were recently invited to a special event for courageous children, in which Abby – having shared her story with a local young carers' group she's involved in – along with her Aunt Vicky, won a special award.

Naturally, Mike and I both attended. As, of course, did all the family. Particularly Kieron. BFF.

CASEY WATSON

One woman determined to
make a difference.

Read Casey's poignant
memoirs and be inspired.

Five-year-old Justin was desperate and helpless

Six years after being taken into care, Justin has had 20 failed placements. Casey and her family are his last hope.

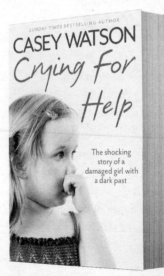

SUNDAY TIMES BESTSELLING AUTHOR

CASEY WATSON

The Boy No One Loved

A heartbreaking true story of abuse, abandonment and betrayal

THE BOY NO ONE LOVED

SUNDAY TIMES BESTSELLING AUTHOR

CASEY WATSON

Crying for Help

The shocking story of a damaged girl with a dark past

A damaged girl haunted by her past

Sophia pushes Casey to the limits, threatening the safety of the whole family. Can Casey make a difference in time?

CRYING FOR HELP

Abused siblings who do not know what it means to be loved

With new found security and trust, Casey helps Ashton and Olivia to rebuild their lives.

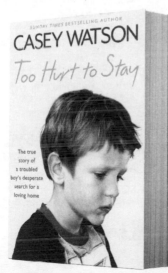

LITTLE PRISONERS

Branded 'vicious and evil' eight-year-old Spencer asks to be taken into care

Casey and her family are disgusted: kids aren't born evil. Despite the challenges Spencer brings, they are determined to help him find a loving home.

TOO HURT TO STAY

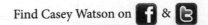

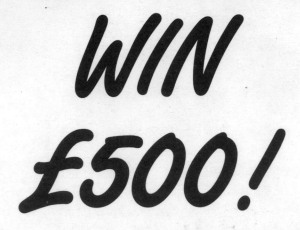

WIN £500!

**'Like' Casey Watson
on Facebook
for your chance to
WIN £500!**

Simply find Casey Watson on Facebook
to enter into the prize draw and for full T&Cs.
PLUS get all the latest news about Casey
and her bestselling books!